Guide to
SKIN AND
HAIRCOAT PROBLEMS
IN DOGS

Lowell Ackerman, D.V.M.
Diplomate, American College of Veterinary Dermatology

Guide to Skin and Haircoat Problems in Dogs
Copyright © 1994 by Lowell Ackerman, D.V.M.

ISBN 0-931866-65-0

Library of Congress Cataloging-in-Publication Data

Ackerman, Lowell.
   Guide to skin and haircoat problems in dogs / Lowell Ackerman.
     p.   cm.
   Includes bibliographical references and index.
   ISBN 0-931866-65-0
   1. Dogs—Diseases. 2. Veterinary dermatology. I. Title.
SF992.S55A23   1994
636.7'08965—dc20   93-37070
                                                  CIP

Cover design by: Robert Schram
Typography: Lyn Chaffee, Amazon Typography

 2 3 4 5 6 7 8 9 0

Printed in the United States of America

CONTENTS

To
my
wife
Susan

PREFACE

Canine dermatology, the study of skin diseases in the dog, has come a long way since its simple beginnings. Today, specialists are performing many of the same diagnostic procedures on dogs as they are on people. And, many of the treatments are the same as well.

Skin disease in dogs tends to be frustrating for owner and veterinarian alike. Many unrelated conditions tend to look alike and the problems are often chronic in nature. It is rare that a simple treatment results in a "cure" for these cases.

Dermatology is an ever-expanding science, and since it encompasses so many other disciplines (e.g., immunology, parasitology, microbiology, oncology, endocrinology, nutrition, genetics, etc.), it is often more complicated than most owners expect. With the explosion in medical information available, with diagnostic testing becoming so sophisticated, and with so many treatment options, it is virtually impossible to be expert in all aspects of canine dermatology. So, it is not surprising that dog owners have a difficult time finding information on specific ailments, how they are diagnosed, and how they are properly treated. The goal of this book is to provide a guide to skin diseases, their causes and treatments, in a format that is easy to read, yet comprehensive.

You will find that the terms used in this book are slightly different from those commonly used in magazines and basic books. Clinical signs replaces symptoms and radiographs replace x-rays. This is because animals don't have "symptoms." Symptoms are those things that people describe about how they are feeling. You may feel feverish, but your dog either has an elevated temperature or not; there is no debate. Since dogs can't speak, they can't have symptoms, only clinical signs. Similarly, x-rays are beams of light of a specific wavelength. We can't see x-rays, but we can see the image they create on special photographic film as they pass through parts of the body. Therefore, we look at radiographs, not x-rays, of patients.

One might debate the need to be so specific in a book intended for the public, but it does impact on our understanding of medicine. Also, it is sometimes disconcerting to owners when medical decisions are not clear-cut, but nothing in medicine is carved in stone. Does a low thyroid hormone test mean my dog has hypothyroidism? No, not necessarily. Did my dog inherit its inhalant allergies from its parents? Probably. My bitch had demodectic mange — will her pups be affected? Sometimes! In this book, we will explore these concerns and many others.

The material in this book is the most current available but, thanks to medical progress, new information becomes available on a daily basis. Don't hesitate to ask your veterinarian for current information on the subjects covered. They are an excellent source for information and likely have more pertinent journals and books than the public library. If you examine the "Additional Reading" listing at the end of the book, you will find examples of current articles and books dealing with the subjects covered. Articles or textbooks that are more than a few years old are bound to provide information that is out of date.

The creation of this book has been a rewarding experience for me and reflects the questions posed by thousands of owners, breeders, groomers, and veterinarians over the years. I hope you enjoy this glimpse into the world of veterinary dermatology.

Lowell Ackerman, DVM

THE AUTHOR

Lowell Ackerman is a board-certified veterinary dermatologist with practices in Mesa and Phoenix, Arizona, and Thornhill, Ontario. He has served on both Education and Research committees for the American College of Veterinary Dermatology, as editor in chief of *Pet Focus* and *Critter Concepts* magazines, and on the editorial board of *Veterinary Medicine*. A graduate of the University of Western Ontario, he obtained his D.V.M. from Ontario Veterinary College. He completed his residency program in dermatology with the American College of Veterinary Dermatology at Cornell University, Texas A&M University, Louisiana State University, and Mississippi State University, and at private clinics in Dallas, Boston, and Cincinnati.

A prolific writer, Ackerman has authored several veterinary and dermatology texts, and published over one-hundred-twenty articles in various professional journals and periodicals.

He is a member of the American Veterinary Medical Association, the American Animal Hospital Association, the Royal College of Veterinary Surgeons, The Arizona Veterinary Medical Association, former president of the Canadian Academy of Veterinary Dermatology and a member of the American Academy of Veterinary Dermatology. He is also affiliated with the Academy of Veterinary Allergy, the Society of Comparative Endocrinology, the Academy of Veterinary Nutrition, the College of Veterinarians of Ontario, the Canadian Veterinary Medical Association, and the Dog Writers' Association of America.

Dr. Ackerman has lectured extensively on the subject of veterinary dermatology across the United States, Canada, and Europe.

1

UNDERSTANDING DERMATOLOGY

Dermatology is the medical study of the skin and the diseases that affect it. In veterinary medicine, it looms large; approximately 40% of all visits to veterinarians are prompted by skin problems. There are hundreds of different diseases that affect the skin, and this often surprises people. The average person may be familiar with acne and psoriasis and a few other conditions that affect humans but not be aware of the multitude of different skin diseases that affect animals. Some are similar to diseases seen in people, and others are unique to the animal world, sometimes unique to a single species.

Not long ago most dog owners thought dogs only got fleas, mange, and seborrhea, but thanks to modern technology and diagnostic testing, those days seem like the dark ages. Today, veterinary dermatology is recognized as an important medical science, often interrelating with other disciplines such as immunology, parasitology, microbiology, endocrinology, oncology, and nutrition.

Like every specialty, dermatology has a language of its own, and the vocabulary is expanding on a daily basis. Older, more generalized terms such as seborrhea, mange, and dermatitis are being replaced by names that are more descriptive, or more accurate. The terms used in this book are very current, but be aware that dermatology is a progressive science and things do change as we learn more. We welcome these changes, because they allow us to better diagnose and treat the dogs that need our help.

1

ANATOMY OF THE SKIN

In dogs as well as humans, the skin is the largest organ of the body. It protects us from the environment, provides a way to conserve and discharge heat, and also acts as a reservoir to maintain water balance in the body. It is the first line of defense in protecting our bodies from a harsh and unforgiving world.

The skin is well adapted to performing its specialized functions. The surface is a tough layer of keratinized (shingle-like) cells that provide a waterproof barrier to the environment. Millions of dead skin cells are shed from this layer each day, and the skin continues to renew itself in an orderly fashion throughout our lifetime. Beneath this layer of dead skin cells are the living cells, the keratinocytes, that live solely to eventually die and provide us with a barrier to the outside world. These cells originate from a basal cell layer, the bottom layer that constantly pushes its offspring toward the surface. The journey from the bottom layer to the top takes about twenty-one days; most cells spend another twenty-one days as dead surface scale before being shed. It is the collection of living and dying cells, that rise from the bottom layers to the top with such regularity, that is referred to as the epidermis.

The epidermis has no blood supply of its own and receives all of its nutrition from the underlying tissue, called the dermis. The dermis is composed of connective tissue fibers, blood vessels, nerves, and a ground substance, which is gel-like and enables the dermis to be firm and supportive yet still flexible. The dermis is also home to several of the white blood cells that guard this territory and provide an immune response when the skin is threatened or attacked.

The boundary between the dermis and the epidermis is called the dermal-epidermal junction, or the basement membrane zone. This zone is very thin, but it does perform a number of critical tasks, including important stabilizing, barrier, and filtering functions.

Beneath the dermis is a large network of fat cells. This area is called the hypodermis, the panniculus, or the subcutis. The collection of fat cushions everyday wear and tear on the skin and underlying tissues.

Hair follicles and the glands that supply them are collectively termed pilosebaceous units. The root word pilus means hair, and the sebaceous part refers to the large grape-like glands that empty their products into the follicles by way of ducts. Production of a hair is a joint venture between the dermis and epidermis. The base of the hair follicle (hair matrix) rests in the deep dermis or subcutis and provides the raw materials for hair growth. In dogs, specialized cells from the epidermis dip down into the dermis before pups are born to form the actual follicle and the "pore" on the skin surface. This is a critical stage, because following birth, no new hair follicles are produced. Since follicles begin as epidermal cells, and since the epidermis does not have its own blood supply, nourishment for the hair must come from the dermis. A specialized structure, the dermal papilla, forms there in intimate contact with the hair matrix to supply it with blood and nutrition.

There are two main types of hair in dogs: the long, bristly guard hairs, and the downy vellus hairs. Whiskers (vibrissae) are specialized sensory hairs that are present in a few choice locations in the body but are not widespread. Guard hairs are sometimes referred to as primary hairs because they originate from the largest and deepest follicles. Vellus hairs, the secondary hairs, are the first hairs evident (puppy fur). They grow in smaller follicles grouped around a primary follicle and share the same opening to the skin surface. Dog fur is therefore described as originating from compound follicles, since both guard hairs and vellus hairs may emerge from a common pore.

There are three types of glands found in skin, and all are located in the dermis. The sebaceous glands are often the most conspicuous; they look like large bunches of grapes located on either side of a follicle. Their job is to secrete sebum into the hair follicles and then onto the skin surface as the hair grows outward. Sebum is composed of cholesterol and waxes. It makes the skin surface water resistant and the haircoat shiny.

The sweat glands of animals are similar but not identical to those of people. Apocrine glands are the major sweat glands in animals. They secrete a form of sweat via ducts into the hair follicle. In people, these glands are present only in the armpits, anogenital regions, abdomen, face, and scalp, but in animals they are present everywhere. The eccrine sweat glands are similar in structure to the apocrine glands, and in people are important in temperature regulation. In humans they are distributed over the entire body surface, with different regional densities, but since they are not used for heat dissipation in animals, they are prevalent only on the footpads and nose of dogs. Thus, dogs do not sweat in the same manner as people and must dissipate heat differently.

THE IMMUNE SYSTEM AND THE SKIN

Part of the barrier function of the skin has to do with the role it plays in the immune system. A special type of white blood cell, the T-lymphocyte, patrols the perimeter of the body, looking for things that don't belong. These T-cells are programmed by the thymus to recognize the difference between the body (self) and everything else (nonself). The thymus (not to be confused with the thyroid gland) is located in the neck and is very large in pups, getting progressively smaller as dogs age.

When T-cells encounter a real or perceived invader, they trigger responses by other components of the immune system to destroy it. An immune system that is perfectly coordinated wards off microorganisms (bacteria, parasites, and fungi) and produces antibodies against many other invaders, especially viruses. However, animals with defective T-cell systems may have problems ranging from recurrent infections to demodectic mange.

In addition to the important lymphocytes, there are other cells in the skin that act in conjunction with the immune system to protect the body. The mononuclear-phagocyte, or reticuloendothelial, system forms a net to catch things that pass through the skin and make sure they get introduced to the lymphocytes. The cells in this system also secrete a number of important enzymes and proteins as well as acting as scavengers by swallowing and digesting things that don't belong. The proteins they produce provide important information to the lymphocytes, giving directions and keeping them updated on what's going on in the body.

Other white blood cells, such as the mast cell, eosinophil, and neutrophil (pus cell) may be located in the skin, and all have a part to play in the immune system's complex balance.

NUTRITION AND THE SKIN

Of all the factors involved with skin problems, dog owners tend to concentrate most on nutrition. People are always asking which dog food is best for skin problems, which supplements should be added to the diet, and which preservatives in dog foods are to be avoided. Clearly, diet does play a major role in health, including that of the skin, but most diet-related skin problems are not what owners expect.

The most important concern regarding diet is that the foods be tested in accordance with procedures established by the Association of American Feed Control Officials (AAFCO) or, in Canada, as certified by the Canadian Veterinary Medical Association. Foods that meet the guidelines established by these bodies are far superior to diets based on National Research Council (NRC) guidelines, which only provide nutrient values that prevent deficiencies. The NRC is neither a government agency nor a research laboratory, and it does not police the pet food industry at all. Since the manufacture and sale of pet foods is a multi-billion-dollar industry, it should not be surprising that many dog foods on the market are there to claim their piece of the action, not necessarily to provide optimal nutrition. To provide optimal nutrition, the food should contain wholesome ingredients and in the proper balance, and be demonstrated by feeding trials to do what it is supposed to do.

Beware of judging a dog food simply by reading the analysis values on the side of the package. You just cannot reliably compare two dog foods by looking at their protein content or by the amount of fat in the diet. Repeated studies have shown that these values are no assurance that the nutrients are of good quality, can be absorbed, or are digestible. It is important to only buy foods that have been tested in feeding trials to prove that several generations of dogs have eaten the food, digested it adequately, and remained predictably healthy throughout their lives. Studies have also shown that some generic and regional brands of dog food (with label guarantees that claim they met NRC recommendations) are not nutritionally adequate for dogs and result in clinical signs suggestive of zinc deficiency or copper deficiency.

Not all foods are created equal; buy the ones whose manufacturers are prepared to provide evidence that they are nutritionally adequate.

As to nutritional supplements, the marketplace is full of them. The fact is, however, that if you are feeding an adequate, balanced diet (tested by feeding trials), these supplements are not needed. In fact, some nutritional supplements do more harm than good. Calcium supplements are notorious for making zinc less available and also for causing bone and joint abnormalities in rapidly growing dogs. Fatty acid supplements are generally sold to add luster to the coat, and although they may contribute to a healthy coat, they may also cause problems. High-fat diets or supplements may actually render vitamin E and other fat-soluble vitamins less available to the body, and they may contribute to digestive problems, including pancreatitis, gall bladder disease, and diarrhea. Feeding a well-balanced and well-tested diet is much more important to a healthy coat than the use of supplements.

Another concern that has surfaced recently is that preservatives in the diet may be causing certain health problems. The preservative singled out most often is ethoxyquin. Ethoxyquin and other antioxidants such as BHT and BHA are added to foods to stop the fats from going rancid. Canned foods have the least preservatives and dry foods the most. The antioxidants allow the food to be stored and maintain its fat content for many months. Without antioxidants, these diets have a very short shelf life indeed. Just imagine how long a bag of hamburger meat would last in your pantry without refrigeration and you can appreciate the need for preservatives.

Preservatives offer convenience, and in exchange, we accept some degree of risk. When you go into a restaurant with a salad bar, there is a very good chance that those fruits and vegetables look fresh (for hours) because they have been preserved with sulfites. Sulfites are generally very safe, but they are not without risks, especially to people with asthma. The flavor of Chinese food is often enhanced with monosodium glutamate (MSG). It is also relatively safe, but it does affect some people adversely. Ethoxyquin is no different — it is generally safe, but some animals may not tolerate it well. How can you tell? If you're really concerned, feed a home-cooked meal to your dog for several weeks using ingredients that are fresh, not preserved. If there is substantial improvement, there may indeed be a diet-related problem that warrants further investigation.

Over the past few years, many diets for dogs have been manufactured and touted as being good for the skin. Most of these diets contain lamb or rabbit, or don't contain soy. They market these diets as though lamb were, in some way, better than other ingredients such as beef or corn or soy. The fact is that these diets are no better for the skin than any other diet. This fallacy no doubt arose because dermatologists often feed dogs suspected of having a food allergy a diet of lamb and rice for a period of time (see chapter on allergies). The diet is fed not because lamb is good for the skin, but because most North American dogs have not eaten it as part of their regular diet. Prior to 1985, very few commercial diets contained lamb. Most were based on beef, soy, chicken, corn, and pork. The important premise here is that you can't be allergic to something you've never eaten before, not that some foods are less allergy-causing than others. If you've never eaten strawberries before, you can't be allergic to them. However, if you are prone, after having eaten them for a while, you definitely can develop allergies. Dogs (and people) can become allergic to foods they have eaten repeatedly, whether it be beef, corn, soy, lamb — or strawberries. Therefore, dogs can become just as allergic to lamb as to beef if they are fed it regularly. This is an important point if food allergy is ever suspected and a hypoallergenic food trial needs to be performed. If a dog has been fed lamb in the past, and many new diets contain it, it is no longer a suitable test diet. In fact, it is not advisable to feed dogs lamb-based diets for that very reason. If a food allergy is suspected, it gets difficult to find something readily available for the diet trial that they haven't eaten before. Things like venison, rabbit, and moose are suitable in these cases, but much more difficult and expensive to find and prepare.

There is also much concern about the soy content of diets and its effects on the skin. Soy is an excellent source of protein and is often substituted for the more expensive meats. There is very little evidence to suspect that soy causes any problems in dogs. Some dogs may not absorb it as well as others; the Chinese Shar-pei has often been noted as a breed with intolerance to soy products. Animals with soy intolerance should not be fed soy-containing products, just as animals allergic to beef should not be fed diets including beef. This represents a relatively small, albeit real, segment of the dog population.

2

ALLERGIES

Allergy, an abnormal response to things in the environment, is very common in dogs. In people, most allergies are caused by substances that we breathe in, that we ingest, that bite us, or otherwise contact our skin. Not surprisingly, dogs are no different.

Allergy is described as an abnormal response, or adverse reaction, because dogs (or people) really shouldn't have problems when they encounter things that normally occur in their environment. After all, pollens and molds have been in the air since the beginning of time — why should they cause problems? Fleas have evolved with dogs over millions of years; why should the bite of a flea be ignored by one dog yet cause another to chew and scratch incessantly? Why do some dogs (or people) occasionally react to things in their diet, such as beef, soy, or milk by-products? Why is it that a shampoo that doesn't bother most dogs cause some to "break out"?

The answers are somewhat complicated, but the facts are that some individuals are more sensitive to some items than are others. Allergies then are abnormal responses to things that the general population shouldn't be reacting to. If everyone got a rash when they ate a strawberry, the reaction wouldn't be an allergy.

A substance capable of causing an allergy is called an "allergen." We refer to that substance then as being "allergenic." Substances that are less likely than others to cause allergy are referred to as hypoallergenic. Hypoallergenic does not mean that the substance does not cause allergy, only that an allergic reaction is less likely.

Individuals that are allergic need only come in contact with very small amounts of allergen to have it cause symptoms. For instance, only about 1% of the total weight of a pollen contains the allergenic portion. That doesn't sound so bad. However, when you consider that a single ragweed plant can produce 1 billion pollen grains and that most pollens and molds can travel thirty miles in the wind, you can appreciate the problem. That's how you can be in the middle of a city where you don't even see plant life and still get allergic symptoms. When you consider that your canine companion has its nose to the ground, sniffing continually throughout the day, you can anticipate the possible outcome.

There is another thing that all types of allergies have in common. As discussed in chapter 1, there is never a reaction the first time you are exposed to the allergen. A dog is not allergic the first time it is bitten by a flea; the allergy develops only after the dog has been bitten periodically by fleas over a period of time. Most dogs with food allergies have been eating the same diet for months or years before a problem arises.

There are also differences between types of allergies. For example, inhalant allergy (hay fever) is more common in some breeds than others and tends to "run in families." Just as it is more likely that if your parents had hay fever, you will as well, dogs tend to inherit the tendency to develop inhalant allergies from their parents. That does not seem to be the case with most other forms of allergy.

INHALANT ALLERGIES

Allergic inhalant dermatitis (atopy, hay fever) commonly causes skin problems in dogs. In the past it has been mislabeled as "grass itch," "grass fungus," and eczema. While humans have mast cells in the respiratory passages that become inflamed and cause sneezing, dogs inhale the pollen but develop atopy in the skin. Dogs don't usually sneeze with atopy; most are itchy and lick, chew, and scratch. It is not unusual that cases are misdiagnosed as flea problems, because the conditions are so similar. If dogs are allergic to pollens, they may have these problems only part of the year, but if they are allergic to house dust or molds, they will probably have problems year-round. To complicate matters further, about 50% of dogs that start out with seasonal allergies eventually have problems all year. Also, most dogs that have a tendency to develop allergies usually develop several. Therefore, a typical allergic dog may have problems with a variety of different pollens, molds, or house dust.

Breeds with a particularly high incidence of allergies include terriers (especially the West Highland White Terrier, Skye Terrier, Scottish Terrier, and Boston Terrier), Golden Retrievers, Poodles, Dalmatians, German Shepherd Dogs, Chinese Shar-peis, Bichons Frises, Shih Tzus, Lhasa Apsos, Pugs, Irish Setters, and Miniature Schnauzers. Any animal, however, pure-bred or mutt, may be affected by inhalant allergies.

Dogs with inhalant allergies usually first begin to show signs between 6 months and 3 years of age, although theoretically a dog of any age can develop allergies. In time, an allergic dog can develop complications such as infections, thickening of the skin, and increased pigmentation. When this occurs, these dogs are often diagnosed as having seborrhea. Any dog with dry, greasy, or flaky skin can be called seborrheic, so this diagnosis is not especially helpful. To best treat the dog, the underlying problem needs to be addressed.

Dogs can do incredible damage to themselves by scratching and biting. The most common sign of allergic itching is chewing at the feet, and the constant licking may stain the haircoat a rusty color. Other itchy areas include the flanks, groin, and armpits. Many animals rub their faces on the carpet, furniture, or other convenient surfaces. The ears are also involved in many cases and the flaps (pinnae) may become reddened and hot. When the skin becomes inflamed, infection is sure to follow, and many allergic dogs develop chronic ear infections or skin infection (pyoderma); the skin also becomes thickened, greasy, and smelly. Self-traumatized areas may develop recurrent bacterial infections ("hot spots").

Diagnosis

Often a diagnosis of inhalant allergy can be made for the dog with characteristic clinical signs and family history. Further investigation is only needed if the allergic season is long, the itchiness intense, or if treatment includes medicines that can't safely be used long-term. If simple remedies such as frequent bathing, antihistamines, or fatty acids can make the allergic dog comfortable, we don't need to specifically identify the cause. Otherwise, sooner or later, we'll need to get to the root of the problem.

Inhalant allergies are identified in dogs much the same way they are identified in people: a variety of substances are injected into the skin and the results are evaluated shortly thereafter. The whole test, from start to finish, takes less than an hour and the results are all available at that time. The testing is often done by dermatologists and may require referral to a specialty center. It is very important that if a dog is to be reliably tested it not be on any drugs that might interfere with the test.

In people, allergy testing is usually done by a series of "pricks" either up the arms or across the back. In dogs, a rectangular area on their side is shaved for the test site and the potentially allergy-causing substances are injected individually. It is not unusual to test for forty or more allergens during an allergy test, so the site has to be large enough to accommodate one injection for each allergen. The procedure is relatively painless, since only a very tiny amount is actually injected, with a very small needle, and only into the very uppermost layers of the skin.

Recently there has been a lot of talk and publicity about blood tests for allergies. Although they do have their place, they are not as reliable as skin tests. Therefore, blood tests with names like RAST (radioallergosorbent test) and ELISA (enzyme-linked immunosorbent assay) sound "high tech," but aren't necessarily your best option. They should be reserved for cases in which a dermatologist/allergist is not available to do more precise skin testing, the skin is too inflamed to allow skin testing, or the owner just won't allow the dog to have its side shaved for the test. When you consider that skin testing by an expert is more precise, allows for better treatment, and is often less expensive than blood tests, it makes sense to opt for skin testing over blood testing if you have the choice.

Treatment Options

Once the diagnosis of inhalant allergy has been made, there are still many options and choices. The goal is to make the dog more comfortable while not complicating the picture too much with drugs. Allergies can be chronic, life-long conditions, and while "masking" the problem with drugs may be convenient in the short term, it can be potentially dangerous over the long term. Because inhalant allergies in dogs (and people) may cause a variety of nuisance symptoms but don't otherwise affect general health, it is important not to use drugs long-term that will trade a "safe" allergic condition for a more serious drug-induced affliction down the road.

SYMPTOMATIC THERAPY   One of the quickest ways to comfort an allergic dog is with a cool bath. The effect doesn't last long, but it does help to relieve itchiness. Be sure the bath water is cool rather than hot, since hot water can actually make the itchiness worse. Adding colloidal oatmeal powder or epsom salts to the bath water makes it even more soothing, and a variety of medicated shampoos available from veterinarians will also improve the situation. It is unlikely that a medicated bath will reduce itchiness for more than a couple of days, but it is a safe way to give your allergic dog some relief, and it can be repeated frequently.

Many allergic dogs have surface infections on their skin or in their ears, and if this is the case, the infections are also itchy. If necessary, your veterinarian will prescribe an antibiotic and/or antiseptic shampoo to treat the infection and thereby also help control the itching. Unless the allergy is being controlled, however, the infection will return once the antibiotic has been discontinued.

Be cautious with medicated creams and ointments, because many contain cortisone-like substances that can be harmful. Check with your veterinarian before using these products. There are many safe sprays available that can give your pet relief. Many contain hamamelis (witch hazel) in a pH-balanced solution (e.g., Dermacool) and/or safe cortisone products (e.g., Cortispray) that can be used safely and frequently for long periods of time.

IMMUNOTHERAPY Immunotherapy (allergy shots, hyposensitization, desensitization) is one of the best treatment options for allergic dogs, as it is for people. The main advantage is that it is very safe, since the shots consist of the items to which the dog has been found allergic on allergy tests. Allergy shots are not drugs. The injections are given according to a schedule and serve to increase the tolerance of dogs so they become less sensitive to their allergies over time. The good news is that immunotherapy is reasonably priced and works in the majority of cases. The disadvantage is that because the shots are not drugs, they don't work immediately nor in all cases. It is a slow process, sometimes taking up to a year before improvement is noticed in those animals that do eventually respond. Once the allergy shots have begun to work, they can be given less frequently to maintain their effect. In this way, allergy shots are like vaccinations, but instead of microbes, other things from the environment are injected to build protection.

CORTICOSTEROIDS Corticosteroids are cortisone-like compounds that reduce itching by decreasing the inflammation in the skin. Unfortunately, they don't stop there. If the cortisone effect were only in the skin, it would be fine, but by giving corticosteroids in tablets and injections, all the organs in the body are affected. In fact, it has even been shown that many cortisone-containing topical ointments, creams, and sprays can end up in the bloodstream if the preparations are used for more than a week or so. Since allergies are long-term, treatment choices for them should be as well.

Why, then, are corticosteroids so commonly prescribed? If the allergic season is short or the amount of drug required to control the problem is small, there is probably not much danger to corticosteroid therapy apart from some transient side effects. Most dogs on corticosteroids will have increased thirst, increased need to urinate, and increased hunger; behavioral changes are not unusual and can be alarming. Most corticosteroids can be identified by the suffix "-one" in their names, such as hydrocortisone, prednisone, triamcinolone, dexamethasone, flumethasone, and betamethasone. The safest tablets to use contain prednisone or triamcinolone, and the safest ingredient for creams, ointments, and sprays is hydrocortisone. Drugs like betamethasone, flumethasone, and dexamethasone are some of the strongest corticosteroids available and are not really suitable for long-term use. Long-acting injectable forms of all corticosteroids are also a much less desirable alternative.

Although corticosteroids can sometimes be used safely, alternatives should always be considered. Long-term use may result in diabetes mellitus, decreased resistance to infection, decreased thyroid and growth hormone levels, increased susceptibility to seizures, fluid retention, and deposits of fat in the liver. Because of all of these potential side effects, corticosteroids should be used cautiously, especially in dogs with diabetes mellitus, epilepsy, heart or kidney disease, infectious diseases, osteoporosis, or ulcers of the digestive tract, and in young animals or those that are pregnant.

ANTIHISTAMINES   As an alternative to corticosteroids, antihistamines are sometimes useful in the treatment of inhalant allergies. The major advantage is that antihistamines are relatively safe compared to corticosteroids. The major disadvantage of most of the classic antihistamines is that they can cause sedation and that they don't work in all cases.

There are many brands of antihistamine on the market, and they work for dogs about as well as they do for people. Many people with allergies receive some benefit from antihistamines but not complete control, and some antihistamines work better in some individuals than others. Similarly, there is no truly "preferred" antihistamine for dogs; some will do well on one antihistamine yet get no help from another. It is a matter of trial and error to find an antihistamine that will work. Unfortunately, we only find a suitable antihistamine about a third of the time; the rest of the time they just don't do much to help.

At least three different antihistamines should be tried in dogs before giving up. These antihistamines are available from pharmacies, and while some require a prescription from your veterinarian, some do not. Most of the antihistamines are intended for human use and have not been extensively tested in dogs, but reported side effects are rare. Some of the more commonly used antihistamines are clemastine (Tavist), diphenhydramine (Benadryl), chlorpheniramine (Chlortrimeton, Teldrin, Chlortripolon), hydroxyzine (Atarax), and terfenadine (Seldane).

OMEGA-3 AND OMEGA-6 FATTY ACIDS   Omega-3 and omega-6 fatty acids are natural anti-inflammatory agents that may also be helpful in the treatment of inhalant allergies. They are special fatty acids that are derived from fish oils and vegetable oils and appear to be helpful in perhaps 20% of allergic dogs. The omega-3 fatty acids are found in fish oils (especially krill and cod), and omega-6 fatty acids are derived from plants containing gamma-linolenic acid (GLA). Important sources of gamma-linolenic acid include evening primrose oil, borage oil, blackcurrant seed oil, and fungal oil.

These fatty acids are different from those found in dietary supplements to produce a glossy coat and, although a 20% success rate may not sound like much, they have virtually no side effects. Therefore, these fatty acids are usually incorporated into an allergy treatment plan along with antihistamines and allergy shots to minimize the need for corticosteroid therapy. It should be noted that these products are much more effective at reducing inflammation than itchiness. Therefore, dogs on these products often have fewer sores even if their itchiness has not been dramatically lessened. Products that contain both omega-3 and omega-6 fatty acids are available from veterinarians. Omega Pet (Bio Catalyst Resources), Derm Caps (DVM), and EFA-Z Plus (Allerderm/Virbac) are prominent brands.

ENVIRONMENTAL CONTROL   Unfortunately, although we always imagine we can keep our dogs away from things they are allergic to, this is rarely possible. We can't keep them in a bubble, but there are certain things we can do to help. For pollen allergies, keeping the animal indoors most of the day is partially effective. Though air conditioners do little to remove airborne allergens, they do limit pollen exposure because the doors and windows are kept closed. Humidifiers, vaporizers, dehumidifiers, and air conditioners may develop growths of mold and should be periodically cleaned.

Many mold-allergic dogs are worse at night, but there are usually just as many molds inside the house as outside. Low-lying properties or those near lakes or marshes have high mold counts, as do homes with damp, dark basements. Adequate ventilation is essential to prevent mold growth in basements, attics, or roof crawl spaces. Also, homes with lots of plants tend to have lots of mold. If your pet is allergic to molds but you aren't prepared to get rid of your plants, consider covering the soil surface with aquarium tank filter charcoal bits.

Molds are also present in pillows and mattresses, as is house dust. If you use bedding for your dog and he is allergic to molds and/or house dust, use synthetic materials and launder the bedding frequently. Kapok, feathers, wool, and horsehair should be avoided as bedding materials.

It is impossible to completely eradicate house dust from a home, but you should be aware that the allergenic culprit is actually a little mite rather than the dust itself. This mite is microscopic, looks like a crab, and thrives at relative humidities of 60% and more. Rooms with carpeting, furniture stuffed with natural fibers, houseplants, and pets are likely to harbor the most house dust mites.

Because a home heating and cooling system can trap much dust, ducts and filters should be periodically cleaned. Activated charcoal filters are best at clearing odors from cooking, foods, smoke, and pets, but by themselves they are less helpful for pollens and molds; they are very helpful when installed with other filters, in tandem. Electrostatic filters help reduce the amount of dust in the air by about 80% but cannot produce a dust-free environment. In addition, they produce ozone, which may cause headaches in some individuals. High-efficiency particulate air (HEPA) filters can clear over 95% of pollens, molds, yeasts, bacteria, and viruses in the air, and when coupled with a charcoal filter can remove most of the dust.

In an attempt to rid a home of dust, keep in mind that many canister and cylindric types of vacuum cleaner actually allow much dust to return to room air as it passes through the bag. Many newer models, including water-trap vacuum cleaners, properly vented central vacuum cleaners, and dust-impermeable liners for standard vacuums have greatly improved our ability to limit dust in the home environment.

Prevention

Because allergies "run in families" rather than having a specific mode of inheritance, prevention is not clear-cut. Prevention must be based on not breeding allergic dogs, but allergic dogs may not show symptoms for several years and therefore may be used for breeding before the allergies become apparent. Furthermore, if the dog is incorrectly diagnosed as having seborrhea, eczema, or pyoderma, the correct cause may remain unknown. Some recent research in people has shown that children of allergic parents, supplemented with omega-6 fatty acids, may actually become less allergic as they grow up. This has not been confirmed in humans and no research has been done to date in dogs.

FLEA ALLERGY

Flea allergy, also known as flea bite hypersensitivity, is a heightened reaction to flea bites. The reaction is not to the fleas themselves but to proteins present in their saliva, which get injected when they bite a dog. Clearly, not all dogs with fleas have flea allergy. In fact, dogs that continually have fleas almost never have flea allergy. The dogs most at risk are allergy-prone breeds that are periodically exposed to fleas. This may seem hard to believe, but it's true. Don't expect the flea-allergic dog to necessarily be crawling with fleas. There's a good chance that you'll never see a flea on a truly flea-allergic dog! You don't have to—once the flea has made its bite, the damage has been done. Even if it hops off the dog, the allergic reaction will persist for another five to seven days. Since the bite of one flea every five to seven days will cause a continual problem in a flea-allergic dog, and since for every flea you see on the dog, there are likely 100–300 nearby that you don't see, you can appreciate the difficulty of managing a flea allergy.

To confirm that a dog is allergic to fleas, an allergy test with flea antigen can be done. This test needs to be read in fifteen minutes and again in forty-eight hours and should reveal a positive reaction if the dog is truly flea allergic.

Unfortunately, using flea antigen in allergy shots is not effective in most cases. Dogs are allergic to flea saliva, and the commercial preparations available consist of ground-up flea parts. How much actual flea saliva do you think is in each vial? Still, sometimes these allergy shots do work, and they are worth trying before resorting to harsher long-term options. When continued scientific research produces a purified flea saliva extract, immunotherapy for flea allergy will be a more rational approach. See chapter 4 for more information on fleas and flea control.

FOOD ALLERGIES AND FOOD INTOLERANCE

It should come as no surprise that some dogs react adversely to certain foods. Sometimes they vomit, sometimes they get diarrhea, and sometimes they develop itchy lesions or hives. Problems due to diet often go unsuspected, because the same food may have been fed for months or years without problem. Many cases of food allergy go undiagnosed and unmanaged because owners refuse to believe their dog could become allergic to the diet they have been feeding without problems for years. Unless the scratching happens at mealtime only, which it almost never does, the connection often never gets made. Another common misconception is that a food allergy can only occur if you are feeding a poor diet. After all, what dog would be allergic to an expensive premium food? The fact is that if you are allergic to beef, it really doesn't matter whether you eat a hamburger from a fast-food restaurant or an expensive steak from a high-class restaurant; you are allergic to the same ingredient. Dogs are no different.

Most reactions to foods cause itchiness rather than diarrhea. In an itchy dog, it becomes extremely difficult to tell the difference between food allergy, inhalant allergy, and the effect of fleas, ticks, or mites just by looking. Occasionally, food-allergic pets will have additional symptoms, such as anal itch, flatulence, sneezing, asthma-like conditions, behavioral changes, or seizures, but these are rare. One helpful clue is that the majority of food-allergic dogs have problems year-round. It would be hard to justify a diagnosis of food allergy if the problems only occurred in the autumn (unless a certain food was only fed during that season). Otherwise, it is just impossible to make the diagnosis by examination only.

Food allergy is a term that is commonly used, but more correctly the problem should be called an adverse food reaction. We don't actually know what percentage of adverse food reactions are allergic. We do know that many adverse food reactions are really a case of "intolerance." Some dogs can't tolerate milk, soy, or preservatives, and this has nothing to do with allergy. Schnauzers may not be able to handle fat in the diet because of hyperlipoproteinemia, German Shepherd Dogs may be prone to pancreatic insufficiency, and Irish Setters may have wheat-sensitive enteropathy. So, even though we're using the term "food allergy," be aware that not every food-induced problem is caused by an allergic reaction.

Fortunately, food allergies only account for about 10% of all allergies, so they are not as common as inhalant allergies. On the other hand, food allergies are much easier to treat than inhalant allergies, so it is definitely worthwhile to test for them if there is a possibility they could be involved.

Diagnosis

It is important to remember that commercial diets contain a large number of different ingredients and that animals react adversely to individual components (e.g., beef, chicken, soy, milk, corn, wheat, etc.) rather than the diet itself. As mentioned above, food allergies are not likely to be worsened at mealtime, and, most commonly, the diet may be one that has been fed for months or years without problem.

A frequently made mistake is changing brands of dog food as a diagnostic test. The most common causes of food allergies are beef, pork, chicken, milk, whey, eggs, fish, corn, soy, and preservatives. Since at least some of these ingredients are present in most commercial dog foods, merely changing brands or types of food may not eliminate the source of the problem. This only works if you are lucky enough to change to a food that does not include the allergy-causing ingredient.

There is no easy way to prove a food allergy. The best way is with a hypoallergenic diet trial. The goal is to feed a diet, for a minimum of four weeks, to which the dog will not be allergic. If the dog's condition improves, this points to a problem in the diet. If improvement is not seen, the problem is unlikely to be food-related. The intention is not to keep the dog on the hypoallergenic diet forever but only to determine if the problem is indeed related to diet so that further action can be taken.

There are many misconceptions about what should be included in a hypoallergenic diet trial. A diagnosis cannot be made by switching from one commercial diet to another. As noted in chapter 1, a diagnosis cannot be made by feeding a commercial "hypoallergenic" diet just because it contains lamb, rabbit, or venison. The diet must be homemade, fed for at least four weeks, and contain ingredients the dog has never eaten.

Any suitable protein source may be mixed with rice and/or potatoes to create a hypoallergenic meal. The meal is prepared by mixing one part lamb, rabbit, or venison (or other protein source to which the dog has never been exposed) with two parts rice and/or potatoes. All ingredients should be served boiled and fed in the same total volume as the pet's normal diet. Once cooked, the meal can be packaged in individual portions, frozen, and then thawed as needed. This diet is not to be fed long-term. It is not nutritionally balanced to be a regular diet. It is only fed for one to two months as a test diet.

During the trial, only hypoallergenic foods and fresh, preferably distilled water must be fed. Absolutely nothing else must be fed, such as treats, snacks, vitamins, chew toys, or even flavored heartworm preventive tablets. Access must also be denied to food and feces of other dogs and cats in the household. Although this is clearly not a fun job, it is the only way to reliably identify adverse reactions to foods.

There are alternatives that seem a lot easier, but don't be fooled. Although blood tests using RAST and ELISA technologies sound like the easy way to diagnose a food allergy, they can be very misleading, since the results are often quite inaccurate. Similarly, skin testing, which is very accurate for diagnosing inhalant allergies, is just not helpful most of the time for diagnosing food allergies. So the hypoallergenic diet is currently the best test we have.

Management

If an animal improves greatly during the hypoallergenic diet trial, the regular diet should be fed for a few days to make sure the improvement was not coincidental. If the problem was food-related, the symptoms should recur within a few days; if the improvement was a coincidence, changing the food back to the original should not make a difference.

But once a relationship of diet to problem has been confirmed, there are many options. For convenience, many owners of dogs with diet-related problems choose commercially available lamb, rabbit, venison, or egg-based diets. Commercial hypoallergenic diets not only contain few allergenic foodstuffs but are also nutritionally balanced. Approximately 80% of dogs with documented adverse food reactions can be maintained on these commercial diets. The fact that 20% cannot is further proof that these diets are not suitable for the testing process.

If you have the patience, you can find an appropriate diet with some further testing. This can be accomplished by adding one new food item each week to the hypoallergenic diet. Fortunately, people and animals with food hypersensitivities usually have reactions to only one or a few substances. Individual foodstuffs (e.g., beef, liver, pork, chicken, fish, corn, soy, wheat, milk, egg) can be added (one at a time) to the hypoallergenic diet for five to seven days, and if they fail to cause a problem, it can be assumed they are tolerated by the dog. If there are any adverse reactions, it is not necessary to continue for five to seven days; the ingredient can be discontinued immediately and labeled as a culprit. If an adverse reaction is noted to any particular ingredient, the challenge can be temporarily discontinued, the animal put back on the hypoallergenic diet alone, the food listed as an "offender," and the challenge continued. For example, if an animal responds well to the hypoallergenic diet trial, one might consider adding some chicken to the diet for a week. If the dog tolerates this, identify some chicken-based dog foods and note their other ingredients. By introducing other ingredients from chicken-based commercial foods for a week or so each, one can determine which commercial food will be hypoallergenic for that particular animal.

Prevention

Fortunately, food allergies do not seem to be inherited in the same fashion as inhalant allergies. However, be aware that some animals with intolerances, such as German Shepherd Dogs, Irish Setters, Schnauzers, and Chinese Shar-Peis may have problems with food (nonallergic) that they can pass on to future generations.

CONTACT DERMATITIS

Because dogs have a fairly dense haircoat, allergic contact dermatitis is not a common problem, since a contact allergen must actually contact the skin (not just the haircoat) to cause a problem. The substances that cause contact allergy are themselves too small to be allergenic, but are absorbed by and interact with the skin to become allergens. Substances that have been reported to cause contact allergies in the dog include plants, topical medications, natural fibers, leather, disinfectants, carpet deodorizers, cement, and plastics. The areas most commonly affected are the abdomen and muzzle areas where the haircoat is the thinnest.

The diagnosis of contact allergies in dogs is not simple, because the test kits made for people are not especially appropriate for dogs. The diagnostic test for contact allergies is referred to as a "patch" test because, unlike testing for inhalant allergies, suspected environmental allergens must be applied to the skin surface under a gauze or cloth patch for forty-eight hours. Obviously this form of testing is not appreciated by dogs, their owners, or the veterinarians performing the test. Some commercially available contact allergens that have been found to affect dogs include carba rubber mix, thiuram mix, epoxy resin, mercapto rubber mix, nickel sulfate, and colophony. Samples of other potential allergens (e.g., ground cover, carpet fibers) must be collected from home and supplied for the test.

Much more common than allergic contact dermatitis is irritant contact dermatitis. This is caused by a large variety of substances that might make contact with the skin and cause "irritation" rather than allergy. Animals with sensitive skin especially may be affected by many products including shampoos, detergents, disinfectants, and salt on roadways in winter.

The treatment of all forms of contact dermatitis is the same—avoid the substances that are causing the problems. Small amounts of topical or oral corticosteroids may help relieve some of the inflammation initially but are a poor choice for long-term therapy. Gentle cleansing of the skin with a mild, hypoallergenic shampoo will help remove the offending substances from the skin surface.

DRUG ERUPTION

Drug eruption refers to any skin problem that results from taking medications. Although relatively rare in dogs, problems have occurred from taking antibiotics, antifungals, antiparasitic agents, vaccines, hormones, topical preparations, tranquilizers, anticancer drugs, and others. In fact, any medication can result in a drug eruption.

Diagnosis of drug eruption is not easy and may be confused with parasites, bacterial or fungal infections, allergies, immune-mediated disorders, and nutritionally related diseases. Even some cancers can be confused with drug eruption.

Like food allergy, the problem may crop up after the medication is given for days or even years, and so a clear association is often not made. A drug eruption can even occur days after the medication has been discontinued.

The rational approach is to only use medications that are clearly needed. Do not medicate your own dog with over-the-counter preparations and keep him healthy with routine care rather than only taking him to the veterinarian when he's sick. Remember, drug eruptions don't occur because the medications are themselves dangerous. They can occur as a sort of "allergic" reaction to any medication given repeatedly, regardless of how safe.

3

BACTERIAL AND FUNGAL INFECTIONS

Neither our skin nor that of our dogs is sterile; it is teeming with microscopic life, including bacteria and fungi. The skin forms a barrier between our internal organs and the outside world, keeping these living intruders on the surface and the outer portions of the hair follicles while the deeper structures remain germ-free.

BACTERIAL INFECTIONS

Pyoderma literally means "pus-producing infection of the skin," but loosely is used to describe any bacterial skin infection. Pyoderma is a common diagnosis in dogs, but the term itself doesn't mean much, because there is usually an underlying cause for the problem. Treatment may be attempted with a variety of potent antibiotics, but if the underlying disorder is not identified and corrected, treatment is likely to be long-term and less than perfect. If a dog has "pyoderma," you've only just begun the diagnostic process; the important question to ask is "Why?"

The most common bacterium associated with pyoderma is *Staphylococcus intermedius,* and therefore most infections are referred to as "Staph pyoderma." It is important to realize that this microbe is present on normal animals and is not contagious. Thus, animals that have a problem with this organism likely have another underlying problem that allows the microbes to flourish on the skin surface.

Common underlying causes for pyoderma are allergies, problems with the immune system, or keratinization defects in which excess scaling on the skin surface gives the bacteria things to feed on. Allergies are by far the most common cause for recurrent infections. Very deep infections, however, often reflect a problem with the immune system.

Diagnosis of pyoderma appears straightforward—why not just culture the skin and see what grows? Unfortunately, there are normally all kinds of bacteria on the skin surface, including "Staph," and just because something grows doesn't mean it's the root of the problem.

Chronic, recurring skin infections require careful veterinary examination, and if long-term, a referral to a dermatology specialist. Many tests may be needed to try to uncover the real problem. This is not always an easy task, because anything that affects the immune system can make an animal more prone to infections.

Pyoderma is frequently treated with antibiotics and medicated shampoos. If the cause was something transient, this may be sufficient. If, however, the condition returns when the antibiotic has been discontinued, it's going to take some detective work to figure out what's going on.

Superficial Pyodermas

Superficial pyodermas are bacterial infections that only affect the upper-most parts of the skin. This classification includes pyotraumatic dermatitis (hot spots), juvenile pustular dermatitis (impetigo), and skin fold pyodermas.

Hot spots are very common infections in dogs. The underlying causes for hot spots include allergies, ear infections, irritated anal sacs, grooming problems, and a host of other possibilities. These infections look raw, deep, and painful, but are actually not deep at all and eventually heal without scarring. Hot spots often surprise owners by appearing to spring from nowhere within just a few hours. They should first be treated by shaving the area so that the infection does not spread further. When the hair is clipped it is easy to see the margin of the infection and normal skin beyond. The treatment most often used is a mild water-based astringent or antiseptic; occasionally antibiotics and cortisone may be needed, but not in all cases. It is not a good idea to apply ointments or creams to the infected areas, because this serves to seal in the infection.

Juvenile pustular dermatitis is also called impetigo or puppy pyoderma and is seen as crops of pimples on the belly of young pups. The term impetigo is not a good one, because that condition in children is a contagious one, and clearly juvenile pustular dermatitis is not. The condition responds well to seven to ten days of antiseptic scrubs of the infected area. Occasionally a short course of antibiotics is also worthwhile.

Fold pyodermas occur in dogs that have wrinkles. The pockets formed in these folds are moist and a great place for bacteria to grow. There are many different varieties of folds, such as whole-body folds in Chinese Shar-peis, facial folds in Pugs, lip folds in spaniels, vulvar folds in older bitches, and tail folds in Boston Terriers. Animals that have folds need to have them regularly cleaned with a mild antiseptic. The only other way to cure the situation is to surgically stretch the fold so that it no longer exists to harbor bacteria. However, most people select a breed for its appearance, including the skin folds, and are reluctant to surgically alter that appearance to correct a superficial bacterial skin disease.

Intermediate Pyodermas

Intermediate pyodermas refer to skin infections that are deep enough to compromise the hair follicles (folliculitis). They are usually easy to see on the belly, where they form little red spots, bumps, pimples, and rings. Eventually, the skin will turn dark in patches because of the inflammation there, and there will be bald regions where the hair has fallen out of the infected follicles. When the rings are seen, many owners mistake this for ringworm. In fact, if you see rings on a dog, bacterial infections are much more likely than is ringworm.

Intermediate pyodermas will not usually clear up without antibiotics, because the infection is deep enough that antiseptics won't reach that far down in the skin. In these cases, a reasonable course of antibiotics is two to eight weeks, depending on how deep the infection goes. If the condition clears up with the antibiotics only to recur once the drugs are finished, then the true cause of the problem was not detected and corrected. It is important not to discontinue the antibiotics too soon, or resistance is likely. Treatment should always continue until at least ten days past the time when the condition appears to be cured.

Deep Pyodermas

Deep pyodermas result when bacterial infections go deeper than the hair follicles. Three of the main terms used to describe deep pyodermas are furunculosis, cellulitis, and abscesses. Furunculosis results when infected hair follicles rupture and release their contents into the surrounding dermis. Cellulitis refers to a deep bacterial infection that spreads between tissue planes and fails to head up into an abscess. Abscesses are deep pyodermas that do come to a head and are full of pus. German Shepherd Dogs appear to be particularly susceptible to furunculosis and cellulitis; an inherited tendency is suspected but has not yet been proven.

Deep pyodermas are serious conditions that may require many weeks or months of antibacterial therapy. More potent antibiotics, such as oxacillin, trimethoprim-sulfa, amoxicillin-clavulanate, and the cephalosporins, are often needed to penetrate into the deeper tissues involved. Antibiotic resistance is common. In the case of abscesses, surgical drainage and the use of hot compresses are first used before antibiotics are started.

Culture and sensitivity tests should always be performed with chronic (long-lasting) or deep bacterial infections. Successful treatment depends on identifying and eliminating the underlying cause. If this cannot be accomplished, long-term antibacterial therapy is unavoidable. This is not only expensive but may also lead to resistance and the increased possibility of drug reactions.

Many chronic, recurring pyodermas for which another cause (e.g., hypothyroidism, allergies, parasites) cannot be determined are associated with impaired immune function. Affected dogs cannot keep their surface bacterial population under control. If this is the case, there may be a history of poor immune status, such as demodicosis as a pup, recurrent ear infections, or bladder infections. These animals are immunologic cripples and are unlikely to regain their resistance without treatment, which may or may not be effective.

Unusual Pyodermas

Bacterial granuloma (botryomycosis) is a bacterial infection in which the microbes have been effectively walled off in the skin but not eliminated from the body by the immune system. The bacteria, having been walled off, are protected from an immune response, and deprived of a blood supply, the granuloma cannot be readily penetrated by antibiotics. Diagnosis relies on biopsies in which characteristic lumps (granulomas) are evident. Culture and sensitivity is helpful but misleading, since it may predict that an antibiotic will be effective without taking into account that the drug may not be capable of penetrating the walls of the granuloma. Once the condition is diagnosed, a search must be made for underlying problems that may be interfering with the immune system, such as allergies or hypothyroidism. Treatment is usually surgical removal of the entire lump(s). If surgery is not possible, or not effective, special antibiotics such as the ones used to treat tuberculosis are given, often for many months.

Actinomycotic mycetoma is a rare bacterial granuloma that may result from contamination of wounds by specific bacteria (*Nocardia, Actinomyces, Streptomyces*). These organisms are not considered contagious to people or other animals. They result in lumps, abscesses, cellulitis, draining tracts, and scarring. Gritty bacterial colonies (granules) are often evident in the discharge from the lumps. Diagnosis may require cultures, microscopic examination of the discharge, or biopsies. Therapy is usually attempted with antibiotics, but surgery may be necessary to remove persistent sores.

Atypical mycobacterial infections are caused by species of mycobacteria that are related to tuberculosis or leprosy but do not cause either of these diseases themselves. Some of the common outdoor species of this genus include *Mycobacterium fortuitum, M. chelonei, M. phlei, M. xenopi,* and *M. smegmatis.* These mycobacteria, unlike their more sinister cousins, are mainly common soil and water inhabitants that may contaminate wounds and sores. They then cause lumps that may ulcerate and discharge. Most are found on the legs or belly. Diagnosis usually involves microscopic examination of the discharge, biopsies, and special cultures, since it is necessary to differentiate these bacteria from the related ones that cause tuberculosis or leprosy. The best treatment is surgery, since most antibiotics do not consistently cure the condition. Occasionally, some of the antibiotics used to treat human leprosy or tuberculosis are used if surgery is not an option.

Cutaneous tuberculosis has been documented in dogs and is diagnosed in the same manner as are atypical mycobacterial infections. Most infections are due to *Mycobacterium bovis,* although *M. avium* and *M. tuberculosis* have also been implicated. Since this infection is contagious to people, diagnosis is very important and treatment is usually discouraged in favor of euthanasia. Most public health officials would rather see a dog killed than have it pose a threat to people. Diagnosis is based on pathologic examination using special stains to highlight the organisms, submitting samples to special laboratories for culture of the organism, and biochemical tests of frozen tissues, done by special laboratories.

Non-Pyodermas

There are many conditions in dermatology that are called pyodermas even though they really aren't. Many problems that were believed to be due to infection have been found to be due to other causes, but the original names for them persist.

Acne, in dogs as in people, is not simply a bacterial problem. Certain breeds, such as the Great Dane, Doberman Pinscher, Bulldog, and Bull Terrier, are particularly at risk, but any dog may be affected. Treatment should involve frequent scrubbing of the area with antiseptics such as benzoyl peroxide, alcohol, chlorhexidine, or povidone-iodine; the condition often improves somewhat when animals reach about 3 years of age.

Callus pyoderma is an infection of the hard calluses that develop on the elbows and hocks of some large breeds of dogs, such as the Great Dane and St. Bernard, and on the chest of other breeds, including the Dachshund and Doberman Pinscher. They result from repeated impact as dogs drop onto a hard surface, usually when lying down. The continual trauma drives dislodged hair and debris (including bacteria) into the callus, resulting in infection. Therapy is often only symptomatic and includes weight reduction, keeping the animal on a padded surface, or having it fitted with protective pads such as hockey elbow pads or a padded vest for chest calluses. The best results are achieved when these areas are protected and when antiseptics are used to cleanse the areas affected. Surgery may be considered, but it is not always effective and is often more hazardous than it is worth.

Interdigital pyoderma, or interdigital cysts, is a form of pododermatitis in which sores are found between the toes. The disorder is most common in Great Danes, Bulldogs, German Shepherd Dogs, Boxers, and Dachshunds, but may occur in any breed. The condition may begin in the front feet, then eventually involve all of them. Although the exact cause of these sores is still unknown, it now appears that few if any of them are actually cysts and that bacteria may not even be the primary problem. Many of these cases respond better to anti-inflammatory therapy than to antibiotics. A full diagnostic workup should be performed, because so many different conditions involving the feet appear identical. Diagnostic testing might include microscopic examination of discharge, skin scrapings, bacterial and fungal cultures, fecal evaluation for parasites, biopsies, immune panels, evaluation for thyroid function, and allergy testing. Treatment for an actual bacterial infection often requires therapy for six to eight weeks with an antibiotic selected on the basis of culture and sensitivity tests, and soaking the feet daily with an appropriate antiseptic. In advanced cases, surgical drainage may be required to expose sites of infection. Most cases caused by immunologic diseases respond to corticosteroids or other immunosuppressing medications. Additional research is definitely needed.

Nasal pyoderma refers to a deep infection on the bridge of the nose. It was often blamed on "rooting" behavior in dogs with long noses (Collies, German Shepherd Dogs). The condition responds only poorly to antibiotics. Although the exact cause is not known, immune disorders are often suspected. Since nasal pyoderma is one of the causes of nasal dermatitis (Collie nose), an extensive workup must be done to confirm the diagnosis. Therefore, such other tests as skin scrapings, biopsies, cytologic examination, and bacterial and fungal cultures should be performed. Therapy includes antibiotic treatment, often for three to eight weeks to prevent infection, gentle cleansing with an antiseptic wash (e.g., chlorhexidine, benzoyl peroxide, povidone-iodine), and protection against further trauma. Recovery is often complete with appropriate therapy, but scarring may result if the area is not protected.

Perianal pyoderma, also known as perianal fistulae or anal furunculosis, is most commonly seen in German Shepherd Dogs and Irish Setters and involves the presence of draining tracts around the anus. The lack of lasting response to antibiotics has led most researchers to the conclusion that the problem is not wholly the result of bacteria. Researchers for years have been trying to determine the cause of the condition and have proposed many possibilities, such as overproduction by local secretory glands, poor ventilation associated with low tail carriage, anal sac disease, or hip dysplasia. The problem doesn't seem to be related to a malfunction of the thyroid or the immune system. One thing that is clear is that males are affected twice as often as females. Diagnosis is usually not difficult, but biopsies and cultures are worthwhile to help provide treatment options. Different surgical techniques have been employed to remove the affected tissues with only marginal success. Cryosurgery, which uses very low temperatures to destroy tissue, is often advocated, and multiple freezes may be required. Some surgeons even recommend removing part of the tail musculature or sometimes the tail itself and often removing the anal sacs as well. Because of a suspected hormonal connection, neutering is often also recommended. A more conservative approach is to treat these cases with a vitamin A-related drug marketed for the treatment of severe acne in people. This has also resulted in some successes. No doubt once the condition is better understood, improved forms of therapy will become available.

Staphylococcal hypersensitivity is an interesting phenomenon, since, although it is frequently seen, we really don't understand how or why it happens. The term describes pyodermas that are very itchy. This is not a hypersensitivity like those seen with inhalant allergies and clearly does not really benefit from treatment with cortisone. These conditions are probably best referred to as pruritic pyodermas or pruritic staphylococcal disease, since therapy with antibiotics removes not only the infection but the pruritus (itchiness) as well. About 50% of cases have some other underlying problem such as hypothyroidism, allergy, immune dysfunction, keratinization defects, etc., that can be identified, but the other half present a mystery. The diagnosis is best reserved for infections that are itchy and in which the itch disappears completely with antibiotics—the use of cortisone at the same time is to be discouraged since it just confuses the issue. Biopsies can be helpful, and an "allergy test" using bacterial extracts also helps confirm the diagnosis. The test is performed by injecting the bacterial extract into the skin and observing the site in 24–72 hours, just like a test for tuberculosis. The best treatment option is to identify any underlying problems and correct them. If no underlying problems can be found, treatment is likely to be long-term, possibly lifelong. Many animals with this condition are kept on antibiotics indefinitely, but this is not usually a desirable solution. About 50–65% will benefit from the use of immune stimulants. These may be in the form of oral preparations or injections with bacterial extracts (similar to allergy shots).

Selecting an Appropriate Antibiotic

When veterinarians select antibiotics for treating skin infections, there are certain guidelines that need to be considered. Since most infections need to be treated for many weeks or even months, antibiotics that can be toxic with long-term use are obviously not a good choice. This leaves out antibiotics such as gentamicin and kanamycin, which are very potent but can cause kidney damage and deafness with extended use. Also, the antibiotics should be capable of getting into the skin from the blood supply and being effective there against staphylococcal bacteria, which are the most likely to be causing the problem. This leaves out ampicillin, amoxicillin, and tetracycline, which are not of value in most cases. Another important point is that antibiotics may work either by killing bacteria (bactericidal) or by inhibiting their growth so they can be removed by the body's immune system (bacteriostatic); sometimes this is a factor in selecting an antibiotic. An animal with a defective immune system (e.g., a dog with demodicosis) needs a bactericidal antibiotic (e.g., oxacillin, cephalexin, trimethoprim-sulfa) that can kill the bacteria, because its own immune system is unlikely to be of any help. Animals with healthy immune systems can often be treated with bacteriostatic antibiotics such as lincomycin, erythromycin, or chloramphenicol. Finally, any breed-specific peculiarities need to be considered. For example, Doberman Pinschers often have severe problems with sulfa drugs, so this antibiotic is probably a poor choice in this breed.

In uncomplicated bacterial infections, it can be assumed that the usual culprit is *Staphylococcus intermedius,* and such drugs as lincomycin, erythromycin, or chloramphenicol are usually effective. If these antibiotics are not effective initially, bacterial culture and sensitivity tests should be performed to determine the type of microbe causing the problem and the antibiotics likely to be effective in treatment. Samples for culture should not be obtained while animals are receiving antibiotics; a minimum withdrawal time of about five days is necessary. In chronic cases, more potent antibacterials, such as trimethoprim-sulfa, potentiated penicillins, and cephalosporins, may be required.

In any antibacterial treatment it is important to remember that it is very unusual for an animal to develop bacterial infections unless there is some underlying problem (e.g., allergy, immunoincompetence, hypothyroidism). If this underlying problem is not addressed, it is unlikely that the infection will be completely resolved. Antibiotics often must be given for many weeks or months and at the proper dosage to clear the infection. Cutting corners to save money or time usually results in an incomplete response and development of resistance.

For animals that appear to have an impaired immune system, immune stimulants are often used along with antibiotics. Although there are some oral preparations that can help stimulate the immune system, most are in the form of injections. Some are derivatives of the cell wall of staphylococci (e.g., Staphoid A-B, Staphage lysate, Lysigen), some derived from Proprionibacterium (e.g., ImmunoRegulin; Immunovet) or from mycobacteria (e.g., Regressin or Stimune). Oral preparations are available as tablets, powders, or liquids. Natural immune stimulants include thymus gland extracts, dimethylglycine, and zinc. Levamisole is a drug used to treat internal parasites in cattle and sheep but has also been found to "boost" the immune system at specific doses. The products currently available appear to be successful in about 50–65% of cases. Since they all work by different mechanisms, if an animal does not respond to one product, it may respond to another.

FUNGAL INFECTIONS

There is a wide variety of fungi that cause skin problems in dogs. Some are very common, some are potentially fatal, and others are just unsightly. These fungi are classified as to how deep they go in the skin. The term mycosis is also used to identify a disease caused by a fungus, since "myco" means fungus. Therefore, superficial mycoses include ringworm and yeasts that act as parasites on the skin surface, intermediate mycoses may extend into the fat beneath the skin, and systemic or deep mycoses may affect internal organs.

Superficial Mycoses

DERMATOPHYTOSIS (RINGWORM)   Despite the fact that there are no worms involved at all, and that the pattern of infection is rarely one of a ring, dermatophytosis is still commonly known as "ringworm." In fact, dermatophytosis means infection with dermatophytes; dermatophytes (which means "skin plants") are fungi that have a specific affinity for the skin. Not all fungi can cause dermatophytosis. In dogs and cats, three species, *Microsporum canis, Microsporum gypseum,* and *Trichophyton mentagrophytes* account for more than 95% of all cases.

It is helpful to identify these fungi specifically, because that can explain how the dog was infected. For example, *Microsporum canis* has specifically adapted for cats, and they are often carriers, perhaps showing no symptoms themselves. *Microsporum gypseum,* on the other hand, is basically a soil organism, and *Trichophyton mentagrophytes* is normally carried by rodents. If we recover *Trichophyton rubrum,* we might suspect that a dog was infected by a family member with athlete's foot, which is also caused by a dermatophyte.

Dermatophytes can only live on the uppermost dead layers of the skin and cannot penetrate living tissue or survive in areas of severe inflammation. Also, these fungi only thrive on actively growing hairs, so the infection spreads outward (sometimes in a ring) as hairs become compromised and go into resting stages. That's why there are bald patches with dermatophytosis, but the hairs eventually regrow as the infection resolves.

Most dogs are exposed to ringworm fungi, but relatively few animals ever develop dermatophytosis due to colonization of the fungi. The body's immune system is remarkably efficient at warding off infections, but a number of circumstances may encourage colonization by fungi, such as a young animal with a naive immune system, trauma, poor nutritional status, contaminated environmental conditions, or a depressed immune system.

Depending on the state of the dog's immune system, dermatophytosis may cause no problem whatsoever, or else create conditions that vary from hairless patches, to scaling, to an inflamed rash, to actual lumps. The severity of the symptoms reflects the activities of the immune system. Ironically, animals with the fewest symptoms likely have the most fungi. Animals with a healthy immune system often react with inflammation when fungi attempt to colonize. Animals with defective immune systems are less reactive. Even if they are not treated, dermatophyte infections typically clear up on their own over a period of time—generally from eighteen months to four years, depending on the immune response. *Microsporum canis* can live in the environment for up to eighteen months, so any building or room in which infected animals have been housed can be a source of infection for other people or animals. Brushes, bedding, transport cages, and other paraphernalia are all potential sources of infection or reinfection. Fungi have even been cultured from dust, heating vents, and furnace filters.

Fungal culture is the most reliable method of confirming dermatophytosis. It may take as long as three weeks to identify fungi by this method. Most samples are collected by plucking suspicious hairs for culture. To properly make the diagnosis once the cultures are grown, all fungal samples should be inspected with a microscope to see if they are one of the ringworm-causing varieties.

Wood's lamp examination using a special ultraviolet light is a quick test but, unfortunately, the results are very unreliable in animals. The test is based on the fact that some ringworm spores will glow green with this ultraviolet lamp, but the fact is that this test will miss the diagnosis at least 50% of the time. Therefore, although it is a quick test, a negative result means little. If, however, some hairs are found to glow appropriately, they should be plucked and examined under the microscope to see if fungal spores and hyphae are present.

Since dermatophytosis may vary from a mild inconvenience to a major skin disease, treatment depends on a number of criteria and varies with the individual animal. Mild infections are self-limiting and may clear up spontaneously; others are chronic, debilitating, and poorly responsive to therapy. The aim of treatment is to cure the infection, prevent the spread of infection to other animals and people, and decontaminate the environment to prevent future infections.

For localized infections, treatment may only involve trimming the area and applying suitable antifungal creams or ointments. This is rarely satisfactory, however, because most dogs have such dense haircoats and the fungi are likely to be widespread. Good products for "spot" treatment include miconazole (Conofite) and clotrimazole (Canesten). Nystatin, which is commonly prescribed for yeast infections in people, is not very effective against ringworm fungi.

For most dermatophyte infections, it is advisable to clip the entire haircoat as short as possible (since the fungi are located in the hair follicles) and to use antiseptic cleansers twice weekly, working them well into the skin. Some antifungal products used as weekly or biweekly dips include chlorhexidine, lime sulfur, and captan. It is important to treat all animals in the household once to twice weekly for at least six weeks until the problem is controlled.

In Europe, enilconazole (Imaverol) can be used as a rinse in a dilution of 1:50 on four occasions at three-day intervals. It is not currently available in North America.

When stronger measures are needed, oral medicines can kill fungi from the inside out. Griseofulvin is the most common medication used, and treatment must go at least six weeks beyond the time the condition appears to be cured. Griseofulvin can cause birth defects and should not be given to pregnant animals. Ketoconazole is sometimes used in very chronic or resistant cases.

Since animals don't become immune to ringworm fungi, it is important to decontaminate a dog's environment to prevent reinfection. It is relatively easy to kill dermatophyte fungi on hard surfaces. A 1:10 dilution of household bleach will kill these organisms on contact. This is suitable for litterboxes, floors, and walls. Kennels, runs, and cages should be cleaned once daily with a 1:4 dilution of chlorhexidine solution, which is less likely to irritate the skin of animals, although disinfectants that contain chlorine, iodine, or quaternary ammonium compounds are also suitable for cleansing runs and cages if chlorhexidine is not available. Brushes, bedding, combs, and toys should be disinfected or destroyed. All grooming tools should be disinfected with a dilute solution of household bleach or formaldehyde, all bedding laundered, and carpets and furniture thoroughly vacuumed.

These last two items present the biggest problems in disinfecting premises. Fungal spores can survive on shed hairs for as long as eighteen months, so these must be removed from the environment to prevent reinfection. Carpeted areas and furniture should be vacuumed at least once weekly, and the vacuum bag should be discarded after each use. Steam cleaning carpets will not eliminate fungi unless an antifungal disinfectant such as chlorhexidine or chlorine bleach is added to the water. Be sure to check for colorfastness before treating large areas.

All heating and cooling vents should be vacuumed and disinfected. Furnaces should be cleaned by a commercial company with high-power suction equipment, and filters should be changed frequently.

A new compound, enilconazole (Clinafarm), has recently become available in Europe for environmental cleaning of dog kennels, but it is currently not available in North America.

YEAST INFECTIONS   Yeast infections are relatively common in dogs, but their significance has only been explored recently. The most common one causing infection in dogs is *Malassezia pachydermatis* (formerly *Pityrosporon canis*), which is normally found in the ear canals, anal sacs, vagina, and rectum. Because it is a normal resident of the skin, it usually only gets out of hand when combined with other skin problems. When the ear canals are inflamed, for instance, there is a proliferation of yeasts there that normally feed on the wax and debris. Allergies or keratinization disorders may be the complicating factor, or even some defect in the immune process. These yeast infections are itchy and musty smelling and most often affect the ears, face, feet, belly, thighs, and neck. This is seen as redness, scaling, hair loss, and thickening of the skin so that it looks like leather.

Candida albicans, the common yeast infection of people, is relatively rare in dogs. When it does occur, it often involves the mucous membranes of the mouth, rectum, vagina, prepuce, and occasionally, the nailbeds.

Diagnosis is not difficult if the yeasts can be seen microscopically in surface discharges, skin scrapings, or biopsies and can be grown in culture. Just remember that this yeast can be recovered from the ears of about 50% of normal dogs, so culture alone does not confirm a diagnosis. Treatment is usually aimed at the underlying cause, but the yeasts can be treated directly with ketoconazole twice daily for thirty days together with selenium sulfide shampoos. Topical miconazole preparations and povidone-iodine rinses can also be used, if warranted.

Intermediate Mycoses

Intermediate mycoses go deeper into the tissues than ringworm fungi or yeasts but still remain in the skin. The fungi that cause intermediate mycoses are usually harmless, common, soil-dwelling microbes that somehow get "inoculated" into the skin by thorns or sticks or anything that might cause a puncture wound. Therefore, even harmless fungi such as bread molds can cause problems if they get into cuts or sores. This actually doesn't happen often, probably because the immune system is very efficient at finding and removing these microbes before they do any real harm.

Because intermediate mycoses consist of so many "normal" fungi, there are no easy ways to categorize them. Because of this, they are often described either by their appearance or by the names of the fungi themselves. Some general headings include the terms eumycotic mycetoma, hyalohyphomycosis, aspergillosis, phaeohyphomycosis, penicillinosis, paecilomycosis, phycomycosis, zygomycosis, pythiosis, rhinosporidiosis, and sporotrichosis. Most of these fungal infections have similar features, such as lumps that sometimes drain and discharge while the animals otherwise seem healthy. Diagnosis usually requires biopsy and fungal culture. Since most of these microbes are common in the environment, culture alone is not sufficient. In fact, spores of these organisms are so common in the air that they frequently contaminate fungal cultures taken to identify dermatophytes. Many of the mold spores that can cause intermediate mycoses are also responsible for causing allergic symptoms.

Another characteristic of intermediate mycoses is that they do not respond to most drugs used to treat fungal infections. The best treatment, if possible, is to surgically remove all of the infected tissue. The reason is that these fungi create walls around themselves that don't allow the drugs to enter and have any real effect. Sporotrichosis, which is caused by a microbe commonly found in the soil and on the thorns of bushes, is most likely to respond to drugs, and potassium iodide, amphotericin B, ketoconazole, and itraconazole have all been used for treatment. Pythiosis, caused by *Pythium insidiosa,* is not really a fungal disorder but was long thought to be. It is diagnosed in a similar fashion to other fungal infections but does not respond to antifungal drugs. Surgical treatment is best, but use of a "vaccine" and plant fungicides have been used experimentally.

Systemic Mycoses

The systemic mycoses usually affect internal organs rather than being limited to the skin. Systemic fungal infections are very serious fungal disorders that normally occur when dogs inhale infectious spores from the environment. These infections are considered noncontagious, although blastomycosis has been transmitted (very rarely) from dogs to people via bite wounds. Many dogs are exposed to infectious spores, but most do not develop any serious problems — usually they just have flu-like symptoms and recover completely. The exception is when animals are stressed or otherwise have their immune systems compromised. In these cases, full-blown and potentially fatal infection may result. Most such dogs develop respiratory infections after inhaling the spores and then the infection spreads to other organs, including the skin. Therefore, most, but not all, dogs develop coughing as a symptom of infection.

There are four fungi that are responsible for systemic mycoses: *Blastomyces dermatitidis, Coccidioides immitis, Histoplasma capsulatum,* and *Cryptococcus neoformans.* The conditions they cause are known as blastomycosis, coccidioidomyosis, histoplasmosis, and cryptococcosis, respectively.

The organism that causes blastomycosis normally resides in areas drained by rivers in the eastern United States and parts of southern Canada. Dogs (and people) become infected by inhaling spores from contaminated soil. Infection is more commonly seen in younger dogs, especially of the hunting breeds.

Dogs with blastomycosis often have symptoms of pneumonia but may also have problems related to the skin, eyes, and bones. If the saliva becomes contaminated there is a potential concern of transferring the infection to people.

The diagnosis of blastomycosis is critical, and finding the microbe on biopsies or microscopic examination of discharge will confirm infection. Radiographs of the chest and blood tests looking for the presence of the organism are helpful but will not provide an absolute diagnosis in all cases. One blood test, the complement fixation test, is considered positive at levels of 1:16 or higher but is not the most specific test for blastomycosis. The agar gel immunodiffusion (precipitin) test is probably the best blood test currently available.

Coccidioidomycosis, also known as valley fever or oidiomycosis, is typically found in the lower Sonoran life zone of the southwestern United States (California, Arizona, New Mexico, Texas, Nevada, Utah), Mexico, and some parts of Central and South America. Most animals that acquire this infection by inhaling spores recover spontaneously and develop lifelong immunity. Others develop serious infections that often involve the bcnes, internal organs, skin, eyes, and heart. These animals may therefore have symptoms such as cough, lameness, fever, and enlarged lymph nodes. Blood tests and x-rays are recommended for all cases, but biopsies are best, since often the organism can actually be seen in the tissues. As for blood tests, the precipitin test (agar gel immunodiffusion) is usually positive within ten to fourteen days of infection and then begins to wane four to six weeks later. The complement-fixation test is not usually positive until eight to ten weeks after infection and remains high for many months. Thus, early in the course of the disease, the precipitin test is usually positive and the complement-fixation test negative. With early active infection, both tests are positive. Later in the disease, the precipitin test is negative and the complement-fixation test remains positive for many months.

Cryptococcosis is found everywhere in North America and is believed to be spread by pigeon droppings, in which the infective form of the organism that causes it can survive for up to five years. Like the other systemic mycoses, cryptococcosis may involve the respiratory system and spread to the skin, central nervous system, bones, and other organs. The diagnosis can be confirmed by identifying the organisms in tissue samples. Blood tests and x-rays are often less helpful than in the other systemic mycoses but are often performed to provide a comprehensive picture.

Histoplasmosis is most prevalent around the Great Lakes and the Mississippi, St. Lawrence, and Ohio river valleys. Fungal spores may be deposited in the soil by contaminated droppings of birds and bats. As it does in the other systemic mycoses, infection occurs by breathing in spores. This is relatively common, and only a small percentage of dogs actually develop severe infection. There are two main forms of the disease; the most common is chronic diarrhea, and the other is pneumonia. Diagnosis requires examination of tissue samples, although blood tests and x-rays are also helpful. Complement fixation and agar gel immunodiffusion are the most reliable diagnostic blood tests. Complement fixation is often used as a quick test and titers of 1:16 are considered suspect and 1:32 or greater are considered positive. The precipitin or agar gel immunodiffusion test also indicates infection.

When diagnosing any of the systemic mycoses, it is important to run other tests to monitor an animal's general health. For instance, it is important to know if the liver or kidneys have been affected by the disease before any drugs are administered.

The most common treatment for all of the systemic mycoses is a drug called ketoconazole (Nizoral). Occasionally other medications such as vitamin C or tetracycline are given at the same time to help increase the effectiveness of this drug. Even then, treatment is often administered for many months to cure the condition. Although most animals do respond to treatment, occasionally it takes years, and not all cases do well. Ketoconazole is much safer than the old form of treatment, amphotericin B, that needed to be given by injection directly into a vein. It was quite toxic for the liver and kidneys and often made animals very sick. Now it is only used occasionally in dogs that are not responding to treatment with ketoconazole.

4

PARASITES AFFECTING THE SKIN

Nobody wants to believe that their dog may have parasites. For many of us, our canines are family members, and we associate parasites on them with uncleanliness. But there are many parasites that prey on our dogs, particularly fleas, ticks, and mites.

FLEAS

Fleas are incredible products of evolutionary magic. It has been reported that the flea can jump 150 times its own length (the equivalent of a man jumping 1,000 feet) and its acceleration is 50 times the acceleration of the space shuttle after lift off.

Despite the fact that fleas have been parasitizing animals for several million years and we know so much about their life cycle, effective control has always been troublesome for dog owners. Owners are always looking for newer and stronger insecticides or miracle flea collars, but their dogs still have fleas if they don't take the comprehensive approach — control on the dog, in the house, and in the environment. It's not really as difficult as you might imagine.

35

Know Your Enemy

If you're going to control fleas, it's important to know a few things about them. They start out as eggs, and two breeding fleas can produce 600 offspring in one month. Most of these eggs are laid on pets, but some fall off into the home environment. Therefore, expect them to be where pets spend most of their time. These eggs hatch in 2–12 days into maggot-like larvae and then eventually spin a white cocoon called a pupa. Don't expect to see the eggs, larvae, or pupae—they're visible only with a microscope. These stages also have something else in common: they're relatively resistant to insecticides. So, when you're spraying insecticides in your home, remember that only the adults are truly susceptible. The cocoon stage can exist for up to twenty months, and then, when the time is right, they hatch into immature adults and start the cycle all over again. If you provide fleas with ideal conditions, they can go through the entire process (egg-larva-cocoon-adult) in three weeks. The adults can live for up to twelve months, but they need to feed regularly to stay alive. Dog fleas will bite people, but they prefer animals; if they don't feed on dogs for two months, they die.

Not all dogs infested with fleas have problems. An animal's flea population is also quite variable, and some may have large numbers of fleas without consequence while others are bothered intensely by the bite of only one flea. Just as some people tend to attract mosquitoes while others don't, some dogs are "flea bags" while others never seem affected.

In a truly flea-allergic animal, the bite of only one flea is sufficient to cause itchiness for up to seven days. Therefore, don't be surprised if you never find a flea on your scratching dog—it doesn't mean that a flea is not causing the problem. Perhaps in some evolutionary strategy, dogs and cats that are exposed to fleas continuously, starting early in life, rarely develop allergies to flea bites. By far the highest incidence of flea allergies is seen in dogs exposed to fleas only infrequently.

Prevention

Regardless of what claims are made by various companies, currently there is no universal flea repellent. The best way to prevent fleas is to keep all of your pets in a flea-free environment. Be aware that it is hopeless to try to keep fleas off your dog if you allow your cat to wander through the neighborhood and then come indoors. Similarly, you can't treat one pet with fleas and assume the others aren't carriers if they don't seem bothered. Once fleas are in your home, your treatment must be comprehensive—don't look for a quick fix.

The best flea repellent to date seems to be a chemical called "DEET." This compound has been incorporated into most human insect repellents.

Because poisonings have been reported in dogs, cats, and people, this is not a product to be used indiscriminantly. The pet product (Blockade, made by Hartz Mountain) should only be used following the manufacturer's directions exactly.

Of the insecticides, pyrethrins, derived from the chrysanthemum flower, are the safest and are also mild repellents. They are present in many flea sprays and powders. On the other hand, flea collars, which often contain much stronger insecticides, do not come close to meeting their claims as flea repellents. They work best when pets don't actually have fleas and may be sufficient control when contact with fleas is only intermittent. "Electronic" flea collars promise "high-tech" flea control, but reliable scientific studies have never shown them to be effective. Also, since the buzz of electronic flea collars can be heard by pets (even though we can't hear them), the sound may bother dogs more than it does fleas.

Some natural flea repellents are available but are not effective in all cases. Natural flea powders are typically made from rosemary, wormwood, pennyroyal, eucalyptus, or citronella. These ingredients can be made into natural flea collars by adding the oils of these plants or their leaves (in a pouch) to appropriately sized collars made from cotton or nylon.

Products derived from citrus pulp, such as d-limonene and linalool, have also been marketed for flea control. A simple preparation can be made at home by adding sliced lemons to a pot of hot water, steeping the concoction for at least twelve hours, and then sponging the solution on the pet on a daily basis as needed. Skin-So-Soft, an Avon product, has been used as a flea repellent and is applied as a rinse using 1–3 tablespoons (15–45 ml) per gallon of water. Using too much leaves the coat very greasy, so moderation is recommended.

Brewers' yeast, thiamin, and garlic have been regarded by breeders for years to be good flea deterrents, but clinical trials have shown no such merit. This doesn't mean that they never work, but they probably don't deter fleas in any predictable fashion.

The natural approach to flea prevention is to be commended, but don't expect that just because a product is "natural" it is completely safe. Poisonings have been reported with the citrus-based products as well as pennyroyal, and virtually any product is capable of causing problems.

Flea Control

To effectively control fleas, you must first understand just what it takes to interfere with the flea life cycle. Your goal has to be to get the fleas off your dog, out of your house, off your property, and then to keep it that way. Flea baths, flea collars, and frequent vacuuming all help, but on their own, none of these will solve your flea problems.

TREATING THE DOG   You'd think it would be easy to spot fleas on a dog, but it usually isn't. A flea comb is a very handy device for recovering fleas from pets and is a very worthwhile investment. Animals suspected of being infested should be combed for several minutes over their entire body, and the material collected should be examined with a hand lens. Not finding evidence of fleas does not mean that they are not causing problems. It is a sad fact that for every flea you find on your dog, there are likely 100–300 fleas in the immediate environment.

All animals in the household (dogs, cats, rabbits, ferrets, etc.) should be bathed with a cleansing shampoo or flea shampoo to remove dirt and fleas. Flea shampoos do effectively kill fleas on contact, but once they're rinsed off there is little residual protection. Don't be surprised if you find fleas on your dog fifteen minutes after the bath — they were waiting patiently and hopped back on as soon as it was safe to do so. Therefore, don't rely on shampoos alone to control fleas.

Dips provide the most complete, longest-lasting flea kill, but they can be toxic and shouldn't be repeated too often. A dip is a product applied to the pet and then not rinsed off. They are usually effective at killing fleas that jump on and bite the dog, but they don't provide 100% control.

INSIDE FLEA CONTROL   The goal inside is not just to kill fleas, but to interfere with their life cycle. Step one is to keep the indoor environment "flea clean." Vacuuming should be done before the application of any insecticides to the carpeting, then not repeated for at least 7–10 days to avoid removing the insecticide. Adding chopped up pieces of flea collar, flea powder, or moth balls to the bag, although this is not a use approved by the manufacturers for these substances, will kill developing fleas within this closed environment.

Step two is to apply a commercial insecticide or borax compound inside to kill adult fleas. Many products will kill fleas, some more safely than others. Seek the advice of a veterinarian for which products are most effective and are safest. If you are using organophosphates or carbamates, it is important not to double up on exposing your pets to these substances by using collars, dips, sprays, and household treatments all at the same time, or you may poison them. (Be careful also of how much exposure you get; if you have several animals to treat, do not attempt to do them all yourself.) Be especially aware of insecticide risks if you are buying products from a pet supply outlet, since you may not be properly cautioned. Consider a pyrethrin-based product, which is safest; the microencapsulated forms will last for about two weeks. An alternative is to add diatomaceous earth to the carpeting rather than insecticide. It is critical that appropriate facewear be used to avoid inhaling this substance.

Recently, borax-based (i.e., sodium polyborate) products have become available that are nontoxic, environmentally safe, and highly effective at controlling fleas indoors. The products (e.g., Rx for Fleas) are added to the carpet, where they inhibit the development of larval fleas, reduce the emergence of adult fleas, and drastically reduce the number of existing adult fleas as well. As a bonus, sodium borate also appears to adversely affect cockroaches. At present, this system works best in households that have at least 40% carpeted floors.

Step three is to kill flea eggs and larvae, which will eventually grow to be troublesome adults. The problem with insecticides, other than toxicity, is that they only kill adult fleas. They barely touch the immature forms. Because of this, insecticide treatments must be repeated every two to four weeks to kill newly hatched adults. Recently, however, compounds have been developed that kill immature fleas and are also safe. These are Insect Growth Regulators, or IGRs. They are insect hormones rather than insecticides; they work by preventing flea eggs and larvae in the environment from maturing further. They won't kill adult fleas, so they are usually combined with insecticides for best effect. As outlined above, borax-based products also appear to directly inhibit the development of larval forms into adult fleas and are thus also important in this stage of flea control.

OUTSIDE FLEA CONTROL   Only certain insecticides are licensed for outdoor use. Most products need to be applied once or twice at ten-day intervals, then on a monthly basis for maintenance. A good strategy is to alternate products, since fleas can develop a resistance to a single product.

The newer IGRs such as fenoxycarb are not inactivated by sunlight and therefore offer some hope of outdoor egg and larval control. Always check labels before using any flea-control product.

TICKS

Ticks are found worldwide and can cause a variety of problems. Because they are bloodsuckers, they can cause significant blood loss in dogs and at the same time transmit many different diseases. Although Lyme disease is probably the best-publicized tick-borne disease today, in different parts of the country different diseases may actually be more prevalent. Ticks can also carry ehrlichiosis (tick fever), Rocky Mountain spotted fever, babesiosis, and the toxin responsible for tick paralysis. Many of these diseases can also occur in people, but they are not contagious from dogs to people or from dogs to other animals. The diseases are spread only by tick bites.

Tick Control

To effectively deal with ticks, you need to understand their lifestyle. In the different stages ticks go through during their development, they usually hop onto and off of a variety of different animals. Most ticks are found on vegetation and are "picked up" by pets and people as they walk by. So removal of underbrush, leaf litter, and thinning of trees can go a long way toward controlling ticks. This removes the moist cover that ticks need and food sources for small animals that serve as their hosts. Careful inspection of dogs and humans after walks through wooded areas and careful removal of all ticks can also be very important in the prevention of disease. Spend extra time checking between the toes and in the ears. Applying repellents (e.g., DEET, Permanone) prior to and during walks through outdoor areas can be helpful in preventing tick bites as well. But insecticides and repellents should only be applied to dogs following appropriate veterinary advice, since indiscriminate use can be dangerous.

In addition to removing the vegetation that harbors ticks, you can apply insecticides to infested areas. Currently only chlorpyrifos (Dursban) and tetrachlorvinphos (Rabon) are registered with the EPA for area-wide control of ticks. Application to problem areas in April or May, then again in June or July, offers the best option for practical yet effective tick control.

Another way to protect your dog is with a new type of tick collar that contains amitraz (Preventic). The active ingredient is not a true insecticide and will not kill fleas on the dog or interfere with flea treatments. It will, however, prevent the attachment of ticks to the skin and will cause ticks already on the skin to detach themselves. One collar will perform this function for up to four months. This is significant, because if dogs wear this type of collar throughout the tick season, their risk of getting tick-carried diseases is greatly reduced. This is because a tick must often be attached for at least seventy-two hours to spread disease, and amitraz will detach ticks within forty-eight hours.

Regular flea and tick collars won't prevent ticks from hitching a ride on your dog, but they can aid in tick control. In most areas of the country, collars should be placed on an animal in March, at the beginning of the tick season, and changed at regular intervals depending upon the insecticide used. Leaving the collar on when the insecticide level is waning invites the development of resistance in insects, including ticks. All insecticide-based collars are potentially dangerous because they perpetually expose dogs to insecticide.

If despite your best efforts your dog does get ticks, he will have to be treated with appropriate powders, sprays, or dips. If only a few ticks are present, they can be "plucked out," but it is important to remove the entire head and mouthparts, which may be deeply embedded in the skin. This is best accomplished with forceps designed specifically for this purpose; fingers can be used but should be protected with rubber gloves, plastic wrap, or at least a paper towel. The tick should be grasped as closely as possible to the animal's skin and should be pulled upward with steady, even pressure. Do not squeeze, crush, or puncture the body of the tick or you risk exposure to any disease carried by that tick. If you're not careful, you might infect your dog or yourself in the process. Once you've removed the tick, make sure you disinfect the site and wash your hands with soap and water. The tick should be disposed of in a container of alcohol or flushed down the toilet. If the site becomes infected, veterinary attention should be sought immediately.

Although ticks tend to congregate in and around the ears, between the toes, and around the head and neck, the entire body should be treated if several ticks are evident. Most dips designed for this purpose are effective, although engorged female ticks may be difficult to kill. Many of the dips, especially those including permethrin, dioxathion, and chlorfenvinphos give some residual protection for up to two weeks. Perhaps not surprising, insecticide impregnated flea and tick collars and medallions are usually not effective in treatment because the insecticide must directly contact the tick in order to kill it.

Unlike ticks that need to live in vegetation, the brown dog tick can infest kennels and runs as well as hide within houses and in the insulation in attics. The brown dog tick has also been found in crevices in walls, in bedding, and in other debris found around kennels. In severe infestations, especially where ticks are located indoors, professional pest control companies should be used.

In kennels, resin-based paints can be used to seal cracks, which prevents ticks from using these crevices while they are developing. Removal of trash in dog runs and changing of used bedding frequently can also keep tick problems to a minimum.

MITES

Mites are small crab-like creatures that can feed on the skin of pets and people. The term mange refers to any and all problems that are caused by mites. Some forms of mange can be hereditary, some are contagious between animals and people, and some just affect animals. Because of this diversity, it is important to consider each of the forms of mange individually.

Ear Mites

Ear mites (*Otodectes cynotis*) cause otodectic mange, and the mites are highly contagious among pets. They spread especially easily when animals are kept close together, such as in pet stores, boarding facilities, and breeding establishments. Despite how common they are, there are many misconceptions about ear mites and how to best control them.

First, many animals can be carriers of ear mites and have no particular problems themselves. Because they appear normal, these animals can be a real factor in the spread of mites; they often go unsuspected when a problem occurs in other animals.

Second, it is not always easy to diagnose ear mites. The diagnosis may be suspected in animals with heavy discharge in the ears, especially young puppies that have been housed closely to other animals. Some dogs will have a dark black discharge in the ear canals that resembles coffee grounds. Head shaking may be pronounced in these cases and damage to the ears may result, especially in dogs with floppy ears. The diagnosis is confirmed by either viewing the mites with an otoscope or by microscopic evaluation of the discharge. In some animals with very few mites present, the condition may go undetected.

Third, the treatment of ear mites is more difficult than most dog owners expect. Mites are quite mobile, and merely squirting insecticide into the ears is rarely effective; the mites simply crawl out of the ears and as far away from the insecticide as possible (usually to around the tailhead) until it wears off and it is safe for them to return. It is therefore important to treat the entire body surface with a safe flea product. Also, all animals in the household must be treated, even if they seem to remain unaffected. Suitable ear drops include those that contain thiabendazole, rotenone, or methylcarbaryl; diluted amitraz is effective as well but is not licensed for this use. The use of ivermectin, either by injection, orally, or in a topical suspension has been found to be highly effective against ear mites but is also not licensed for this purpose. It is sometimes used for stubborn kennel infestations.

Demodectic Mange

Demodectic mange is an important and controversial disease in dogs. The mites that cause demodectic mange (demodicosis) are found in the hair follicles of all normal animals as well as people. Demodectic mange is therefore considered noncontagious, since all animals already have these mites. Apparently, animals are not born with the mites but acquire them from their mothers in the first few days of life, as they nurse. They can also be transmitted from one pup to another during this time.

The controversy surrounding demodectic mange has to do with the possibility that it's heritable. It is currently believed that the only animals that have real problems with this parasite are those whose immune systems are not functioning properly. This could happen from time to time in stressed animals but could also be the result of an inherited or acquired immune problem. In people, *Demodex* mites usually only cause problems in people with immune malfunctions such as AIDS. Therefore, when young animals are affected, we often suspect an inherited immune defect. These are very difficult to prove, however, because at present there is no quick and efficient test of immune status in dogs.

Many breeds appear predisposed to demodicosis, including Doberman Pinschers, Chinese Shar-peis, Boxers, Great Danes, German Shepherd Dogs, Collies, Bull Terriers, English Bulldogs, Boston Terriers, Dalmatians, Old English Sheepdogs, Afghan Hounds, Dachshunds, Beagles, and Staffordshire Terriers.

Not all young animals afflicted with demodicosis are destined to be immunologically handicapped for life. A large percentage tend to self-cure when their immune systems are fully developed. This can happen anywhere from 8 months to 3 years of age, depending on the breed. A dog can't recover if bacteria and mites continually challenge its immune system. However, a dog with a normal immune system, even an immature one, should be able to bring the *Demodex* mite population under control with only supportive care. It is estimated that 90% of pups affected will improve naturally if given supportive care, which might include cleansing shampoos, antibiotic therapy, and immune stimulants. The 10% that do not spontaneously improve should be considered to be immunologically crippled, although they can still be made symptomatically better by using insecticides to kill the mite population. Older animals that suddenly develop demodicosis should be very carefully screened for underlying reasons for the developing immune dysfunction.

Clinically, animals with demodicosis have sores and infections which may be localized or generalized depending on how much their immune systems are impaired. Demodicosis used to be described as "localized" or "generalized" based on the number of affected patches, how big they were, or where they were located, but we now appreciate that the most important distinction is how much treatment is needed to make the pet better. Clearly, the easier the condition clears up, the better the prognosis.

The diagnosis of demodicosis is usually not difficult if the skin is firmly squeezed (to express the mites from the follicles), then scraped with a scalpel blade, and the collected material examined with a microscope. The adult mites are often described as resembling cigars or alligators, and the eggs are more teardrop-shaped. Animals that have thick skin or folds may require biopsy before the mites can be seen.

The treatment of demodicosis depends on the underlying cause of the immune defect. For young animals, it is usually best to wait until the animal reaches immunologic maturity before using treatments designed to kill the mites, unless the condition gets progressively worse. If insecticides are used to kill the mites, they should be used with the assumption that the animal is immunologically handicapped and would not get better on its own. After all, a dog with a normal immune system would not be having problems with this mite. This warrants neutering the dog to make sure it does not contribute to future generations of immunologically disabled animals, but for breeders this can create difficulty. They often don't want to neuter a young dog with mild demodicosis, because the condition could clear up on its own and the dog could be used for breeding. In the interim, they want to start treatment to clear up the dog for show. It is then impossible to determine if the condition would have resolved on its own (good news) or if it would have gotten worse without treatment (bad news). The breeder ends up with a dog that looks normal even though it may be passing an immune defect on to pups.

For dogs, the preferred treatment for generalized demodicosis is amitraz (Mitaban®), which is one of the more effective products licensed for this use. The product is applied as a dip, which means it is worked into the skin and not rinsed off. The dips are applied every two weeks exactly as recommended by the manufacturer until mites are no longer recovered. It is imperative that animals not get wet between dips, or the treatment will be removed from the skin surface. It is also recommended that animals be clipped or shaved so that the treatment can be most effective. Since the mites live in the hair follicles, it is imperative that the dip contact the skin surface and not be soaked up in the fur. Animals should then be allowed to air dry and not be toweled or blown dry.

In general, progress is measured by performing skin scrapings before each dip. When two successive scrapings are negative, the dips are discontinued. There are many misconceptions about the use of amitraz for demodicosis. Some people say therapy requires six treatments, while others might say twelve. The correct answer is that dips must be repeated until there are no mites left, or the mites will eventually repopulate the skin. This may require a few dips or many, and some dogs are on lifelong treatment. The average success rate is about 60%; dermatologists have often extended this success rate to 80% by varying dosage regimens and treatment intervals. Experiments with a new medication, milbemycin oxime, used in some heartworm preventives, have also shown some beneficial results in the treatment of generalized demodicosis. Finally, although ivermectin has not been successful alone in the treatment of demodicosis, combining it with weekly amitraz dips has been recommended for resistant cases. This combination is not a licensed use of either product.

Scabies

Sarcoptic mange, or "scabies," is probably the itchiest condition affecting dogs. The mite responsible is also capable of biting people, although it does not appear to be able to reproduce and lay eggs on them. This mite burrows into the uppermost layers of a dog's skin and creates intense itchiness. The preferred areas are the edges of the ears, the elbows, the hocks, and the breastbone and other sparsely haired areas. Affected areas are constantly scratched, and the traumatized skin is often covered with crusts or scabs.

Diagnosis is sometimes difficult, because the mites are very hard to find on skin scrapings. It is not unusual for multiple scrapings to be done before evidence of the mites is found, and in many cases the mites are never found. Since diagnosis is difficult but treatment is relatively easy, the credo of many veterinary dermatologists has become, "If scabies is suspected, treat for it!"

Although treatment of scabies is fairly simple, there is some evidence of resistance to a variety of products in different parts of the country. All animals in the household should be treated, but humans do not usually require therapy; since the mites cannot reproduce on people, they die out as soon as the animals have been effectively treated.

There are two options when it comes to treatment. Many of the conventional organophosphate insecticides must be applied as a dip every week or two for 4–6 weeks to be effective. The same is true for lime sulfur dips. Flea shampoos are unlikely to be effective. The second option is to use amitraz (Mitaban®) dip or ivermectin injections and repeat the treatment two weeks later. This second option is very effective, but these products are not currently licensed for this use. Amitraz (Mitaban®) is licensed only for the treatment of demodectic mange, and ivermectin is licensed only for the prevention of heartworm disease. The dose of ivermectin needed to kill scabies is approximately fifty times that needed to prevent heartworm. Ivermectin should not be used in Collies because it appears to be quite toxic in this particular breed.

Cheyletiellosis

Cheyletiellosis is caused by several different species of *Cheyletiella* mites and has been nicknamed "walking dandruff." They are just large enough to be seen by a very keen eye, or with the use of a hand lens. These mites do not burrow; they feed on the scales present on the skin surface. They are contagious to other animals as well as people and are more commonly seen in cats than in dogs. This mite, unlike scabies or *Demodex,* is capable of living in the environment for an extended time, perhaps up to ten days.

People can be affected with these mites and therefore diagnosis and treatment are important. Not all animals respond the same way to these mites; some animals may have no signs of problems, others may have dandruff, and others may be intensely itchy. The diagnosis is not as difficult as for sarcoptic mange, although the mites are not always easy to find. They can be collected by skin scrapings, acetate (Scotch) tape, or even a modified vacuuming technique.

The treatment options for cheyletiellosis are the same as for sarcoptic mange.

Chiggers

Trombiculiasis is caused by the larvae of chiggers—the adults do not feed on animals at all. The larvae usually parasitize rodents, birds, snakes, and lizards in wooded areas, but they will also latch onto roaming dogs and cats. This problem is more prevalent in the late summer and fall. The bites of chigger mites are quite irritating and itchy, and most are likely to occur on the head and feet.

The diagnosis may be suspected when dogs have been in infested forests in late summer or fall and can be confirmed by finding the mite larvae. Occasionally the larvae may be seen as orange dots on the skin surface, but skin scrapings are often more helpful. Treatment is not difficult, as the larvae are susceptible to many insecticides, including carbaryl, amitraz, and pyrethrins. Irritation from the bites may persist for several days.

Nasal Mites

Pneumonyssoides caninum is the nasal or sinus mite of dogs, and may result in a runny nose (rhinitis), itchiness (especially of the face), sneezing, and other respiratory problems. It is just large enough to be seen without a microscope and may be found wandering around the nose and muzzle area. Alternatively, it is sometimes seen in samples of nasal discharge or in the nasal passages. Ivermectin is the treatment of choice and quite effective, but it is not currently licensed for this use.

OTHER PARASITES

Lice

Lice are uncommon parasites of dogs, and the ones that affect dogs are not really contagious to people. They might bite people, but they can't survive and reproduce on them. Adult lice and nits are large enough to be seen without a microscope, so diagnosis usually isn't difficult. Treatment is also relatively straightforward, since many flea shampoos will be effective. It is important to treat all animals in the household to completely get rid of lice.

Pelodera

Pelodera strongyloides is a worm that may be found in damp organic matter such as hay or straw. It can be a problem if bedding is made of these substances, so the easiest way to prevent this parasite is not to use hay or straw as bedding for dogs. Treatment involves getting rid of the infested bedding and using an appropriate dip, as recommended by a veterinarian.

Heartworm

Heartworm is a worm that usually lives in the heart and pulmonary arteries, but occasionally the immature forms, the microfilariae, end up in the blood vessels of the skin and can cause itchiness, redness, and even lumps. Diagnosis can be made with biopsies or blood tests, and treatment requires very close veterinary supervision.

Hookworm

Hookworm is a worm that usually is found in the intestines, but one way that people and animals can get infected is by the larvae penetrating the skin directly. They can even puncture the skin through a beach towel. Many of the newer heartworm preventives are also effective against hookworm, but specific treatments can be prescribed if necessary.

Flies

Flies can cause problems in dogs, either by biting them (especially on the ear tips) or by laying their eggs, which later hatch into maggots (myiasis), in wounds. Larvae of the botfly *Cuterebra* can even penetrate the skin directly and grow beneath it, leaving a breathing pore. Fly bites can often be discouraged by applying suitable insecticides or thin layers of petroleum jelly to susceptible areas. Animals with maggots often require hospitalization, surgical trimming of the area and maggot removal, cleansing and disinfection, and often antibiotics. Do not allow animals outdoors with open sores.

Leishmaniasis

Leishmaniasis is caused by a protozoal organism that is spread by sandflies. It is most commonly found in the Mediterranean, but in the last few years pockets of infection have been found (in people and animals) in the Southwest, particularly Oklahoma and Texas. Diagnostic and treatment efforts are quite involved.

Dracunculiasis

Dracunculiasis is a rare condition in which a long slender worm forms a cyst-like swelling beneath the skin. Surgical removal is the best treatment.

INSECTICIDE ALERT

People use a variety of insecticide products in the home and kennel, but relatively few are truly aware of how dangerous handling such products can be. Your health is priceless, and unless you learn about the products you're using, you're putting it at very serious risk. Either have a professional apply the insecticide for you, or make sure you know how to use it safely.

The safest products to use in parasite control are always pyrethrin-based insecticides and insect growth regulators. The pyrethrins may not give you the longest period of parasite control, but they are much less likely to poison you or your pets.

The insect growth regulators are not insecticides and are safe to use in all flea control programs. Most last in the environment for about two months and stop immature forms of fleas from developing into adults, thereby breaking the life cycle. They are extremely safe and unlikely to cause poisonings. Because these products will not kill adult fleas (remember, they are insect hormones, not insecticides), they may be combined with insecticides to give a more comprehensive effect.

Amitraz is licensed for the treatment of demodectic mange. Since it first appeared in the marketplace with almost miraculous claims, amitraz has now been accepted as a useful product but not one that will cure all cases. Side effects are rare but may include sedation, low blood pressure, bloat, and vomiting.

Ivermectin is licensed as a heartworm preventive but has also been found to be effective in the treatment of many other parasites, albeit at higher doses. The product is generally regarded as quite safe but, for some reason, Collies and their crosses are very prone to being poisoned by this product.

The organophosphates and carbamates have a long-lasting effect but are potentially much more toxic than the pyrethrins. They are commonly incorporated into sprays, flea collars, and dips and are fairly stable in the environment, lasting for many weeks. Most poisonings result because people will apply an organophosphate or carbamate dip to the pet, then apply an organophosphate or carbamate flea collar, then use an organophosphate or carbamate spray or "bomb" in the house. They may be following the directions on each individual product but they're not considering the cumulative effects on the dog or themselves.

Table 4.1. Insecticides and Insect Growth Regulators

Class	Generic	Example
Pyrethrins	Pyrethrin	Parid-X; Para mist
Pyrethroids	Resmethrin	Durakyl
	d-trans allethrin	Duocide
	Fenvalerate	VIP
	Permethrin	Duocide LA; Synerkyl
	d-phenothrin	Duocide
	Tetramethrin	Sprecto-CF
Carbamates	Carbaryl	D-F-T; Happy Jack
	Bendiocarb Propoxur	
Organophosphates	Chlorpyrifos (Dursban)	Duratrol
	Cythioate	Proban
	Diazinon	Escort
	Dichlorvos	Vapona; Task
	Dioxathion	Del-Tox
	Fenthion	Prospot
	Malathion	Adams Flea/Tick Dip
	Phosmet	Paramite
	Tetrachlorvinphos	Rabon

Table 4.1. *Continued*

Class	Generic	Example
Insect Growth Regulators	Methoprene	Siphotrol
	Fenoxycarb	Ectogard
Formamidines	Amitraz	Mitaban; Preventic
Avermectins	Ivermectin	Ivomec; Heartgard
	Milbemycin oxime	Interceptor

5

KERATINIZATION DISORDERS (SEBORRHEA)

Few diagnoses are as confusing to dog owners as seborrhea. Part of the confusion arises because most dogs said to have this disorder do not, in fact, have seborrhea. Seborrhea has become a catch-all term for any case of dry, scaly, smelly, or greasy skin, regardless of cause.

Unfortunately, most skin problems that cause any degree of inflammation result in these changes, so that most, at one time or another, can get labeled as "seborrhea." It is one of those words, like dermatitis or eczema, that is used frequently but means little. In fact, the problem can be compounded, because dry skin is often referred to as seborrhea sicca and oily skin as seborrhea oleosa, as though that provides important additional information, and red, inflamed skin may be called seborrheic dermatitis. The problem is compounded further because there is an actual condition known as seborrhea, which is extremely rare in dogs. So seborrhea as a description is phenomenally common, but probably less than 1% of dogs so labeled actually have true seborrhea.

The proper description for this collection of problems is keratinization disorders. Keratin is the scale on the surface of the skin, and all the symptoms listed above can be explained by some abnormality of the arrangement of this keratin on the skin surface. Some arrangements make the skin dry, others greasy, and all can make the skin inflamed. Since most of the problems that cause these keratinization disorders have nothing to do with the sebaceous glands, seborrhea (which means "flow of sebum") is a poor diagnosis most of the time.

Allergies can commonly result in keratinization disorders, as can hormonal problems, nutritional problems, inherited problems, infections, autoimmune diseases, and even some cancers. Some animals undoubtedly are born with a defect in their keratinization process (e.g., ichthyosis, epidermal dysplasia, seborrhea), but by far, most keratinization disorders occur secondary to underlying problems. It is therefore critical not to stop with a diagnosis of keratinization disorder until the cause for it has been established. Treat the cause and, more often than not, the keratinization disorder will take care of itself.

Why do animals respond this way to such a variety of underlying problems? Most people shed millions of dead skin cells into the environment every day, and the dog is no different. The skin is constantly in a process of renewal and there is an orderly progression for a plump epidermal cell to evolve into dead surface scale. This process takes about twenty-one days, then another twenty-one days for the scale to shed into the environment. If some problem disturbs this sequence and scale collects haphazardly on the skin surface, sometimes the scale is greasy in texture and other times it is dry like dandruff. There can be scaling, crusting, and hair loss. Normal bacteria on the skin surface increase in number as they have more debris on which to feed; as they break down the fatty substances in the scale they give off a rancid odor. As the bacteria flourish further, they can cause infections on the skin surface. Dogs often damage these areas even more by scratching.

Diagnosing keratinization disorders properly is an involved process, because so many different possibilities exist. Some problems are more common in specific breeds, and this can help direct diagnostic efforts. In other cases, a step-by-step approach might include skin scrapings, bacterial and fungal cultures, blood tests, allergy assessment, and biopsies. A non-specific diagnosis of keratinization disorder should only be made after all other possible underlying causes have been considered and excluded.

Treatment is very successful when the underlying provoking factors have been identified and corrected. Thus, hypothyroidism can be corrected by thyroid replacement therapy, nutritional problems by dietary correction, infections by antibiotic therapy, etc. For disorders in which an underlying condition cannot be identified, treatment must be vigorous and intensive, though in most cases the animal's overall health is not compromised. These animals may look dreadful, but only rarely is the keratinization disorder associated with internal problems.

Frequent bathing and topical treatment of the skin, as well as perhaps dietary supplementation, may make the condition more tolerable if a more specific therapy is not available. This usually means bathing from twice weekly to once every few weeks with an antiseborrheic shampoo. Ingredients considered antiseborrheic include sulfur, salicylic acid, tar, selenium sulfide, and benzoyl peroxide. One should always use tar shampoos with some caution, since they may irritate the skin and can result in contact dermatitis in the person doing the bathing—always wear gloves when using tar shampoos. Benzoyl peroxide, which is a common ingredient in acne products, can dry the skin and can bleach many fabrics. Therefore, it should not be used in dogs with overly dry skin unless the bath is followed by an emollient rinse or spray. Benzoyl peroxides are particularly helpful in cases where the scale collects in the hair follicles, such as it does in Schnauzer comedo syndrome and vitamin A-responsive dermatosis. For best effect, all antiseborrheic shampoos should be worked into and then left on the animal's skin (not just the haircoat) for 5–15 minutes after thorough lathering, or as recommended by the manufacturer. Proper rinsing is essential, and animals preferably should be air-dried or towel-dried rather than blown dry.

Dogs with keratinization disorders often benefit from a good basic diet, and supplementing that diet with essential fatty acids on a regular basis may help alleviate some of the scaling. These supplements might include sources of gamma-linolenic acid (evening primrose oil, borage oil, blackcurrant oil, sunflower oil) or marine lipids (fish oils), and combination products are available commercially (e.g., Omega Pet, DermCaps, EFA-Z Plus). Finally, some keratinization disorders have responded to vitamin A or its more potent, synthetic cousins, the retinoids.

UNDERLYING PROBLEMS CAUSING KERATINIZATION DISORDERS

As explained above, secondary keratinization disorders are much more common than specific defects of the keratinization process. Most of these conditions are discussed in their respective chapters.

Allergies are probably the most common cause of keratinization disorders in dogs. Inhalant allergies, food allergies, drug eruptions, and contact sensitivities have all been implicated. Even immune-mediated disorders such as pemphigus and lupus can result in marked scaling.

Parasites, especially fleas and mites, can cause symptoms that are hard to differentiate from "seborrhea." Bacterial infections and ringworm infections can also appear very similar.

Hormonal problems, especially hypothyroidism, Cushing's disease, growth hormone-responsive dermatosis, and sex hormone disorders can also result in keratinization disorders, and often secondary bacterial infection. Nutritional disturbances such as vitamin A-responsive dermatosis, zinc-responsive dermatosis, and fatty acid deficiency can cause scaling; even some cancers, especially T-cell lymphomas, can look like keratinization disorders.

Inherited keratinization disorders are discussed in the chapter on breed-related skin problems and usually cause symptoms that are evident by four months of age. Most of the other problems are not evident in pups this young, except perhaps ringworm and some of the external parasites.

Although keratinization disorders secondary to other problems will resolve on their own when the primary cause has been adequately addressed, this doesn't happen overnight. If the problem were instantly corrected, it would still take about six weeks before the improvement would be apparent. This is because it takes new skin cells about three weeks to make it to the stratum corneum and about another three weeks to be shed. Since no treatment is instantaneous, successful treatment usually results in resolution of the keratinization disorder in 3–4 months. Therefore, be understanding and patient; overnight miracles do not happen.

CONGENITAL KERATINIZATION DISORDERS

Most congenital keratinization disorders are evident in young pups and reflect a defect in the way their skin cells arrange themselves. For the most part, these conditions are diagnosed by biopsy, and treatment is symptomatic only. Medications can be given that alter the process, but rarely are these conditions "cured." Therefore, treatment is directed at controlling the situation rather than curing it, and in most cases, therapy will be necessary for life.

Epidermal Dysplasia

Epidermal dysplasia is seen in young pups, most often in West Highland White Terriers. Just as hip dysplasia refers to a developmental defect of the hip joints, epidermal dysplasia reflects a developmental defect in epidermal turnover, the keratinization process. Affected pups are often itchy, their skin becomes dark and thickened, and in many ways they look like severely allergic pups, only younger than usual. These animals are frequently also prone to yeast infections. Diagnosis is made by biopsy, and treatment is very intensive, using topical preparations and strong oral medications. The vitamin A derivatives, especially etretinate, are used to help normalize the keratinization process; bathing with this must be done frequently to remove the prominent scale. The genetic nature of epidermal dysplasia is not yet fully understood.

Seborrhea

Seborrhea (true seborrhea) is also a primary defect of the keratinization process. It is seen in the Cocker Spaniel, Springer Spaniel, Irish Setter, Basset Hound, West Highland White Terrier, Doberman Pinscher, Chinese Sharpei, and Labrador Retriever. Young animals develop all the characteristic features of "seborrhea," including waxy ears and bacterial infections. Research to date has shown that the epidermal cells of affected animals have a greatly accelerated turnover rate, which causes them to collect in a haphazard fashion on the skin surface. There can also be changes in the surface lipids (fats). The clinical picture is also very similar to and often confused with allergic inhalant dermatitis. Diagnosis can usually be made on biopsy specimens. Treatment is symptomatic and similar to that for epidermal dysplasia. This condition is likely genetically influenced, so affected animals and their close relations should not be used for breeding.

Ichthyosis

Ichthyosis is a genetic disease that results in extreme scaling, especially of the footpads, although the dog's whole body is affected. Once again, this is a disease of young dogs, usually quite evident before six months of age. Diagnosis is made by biopsy, and since the problem is inherited, treatment is directed against the symptoms, just as in epidermal dysplasia and seborrhea.

NUTRITIONALLY RELATED KERATINIZATION DISORDERS

Zinc-Responsive Dermatosis

Zinc-responsive dermatosis is a scaling skin disease that is improved by adding zinc to the diet. Note that the name of the condition is not zinc deficiency, because dogs that have it usually have blood zinc levels in the normal range. Thus, these animals have a higher than normal requirement for zinc rather than a deficiency. There are two forms of the disorder, one in rapidly growing puppies, and one with a predilection for the sled dog breeds.

Some ingredients in dog foods, and supplements such as calcium, phytates, iron, tin, and copper have all been shown to decrease zinc absorption, so one of the important causes of zinc-responsive dermatosis is owners giving their pets nutritional supplements. Calcium supplements are major offenders and generally should not be given by owners to rapidly growing dogs. Some members of breeds such as the Siberian Husky, Malamute,

Samoyed, and perhaps the Great Dane and Doberman Pinscher, may have a genetic defect that results in a decreased ability to absorb zinc from the intestine. This may also then result in a greater need for zinc.

Most dogs with zinc-responsive dermatosis have accumulations of scale and crust on their face, elbows, and hocks. It is quite likely that the old condition "dry pyoderma" was really undiagnosed cases of zinc-responsive dermatosis. Young dogs of rapidly growing breeds that have been oversupplemented (especially with calcium) may also have stunted growth, bone deformities, and a poor appetite. The diagnosis is made by biopsy of affected skin, and the changes reported by pathologists are quite characteristic.

Treatment is straightforward and relatively easy. Dogs that have been oversupplemented will respond to eliminating the supplementation and returning them to a balanced diet. Dogs with inherited defects will probably require some form of zinc supplementation for life. This is usually administered in the form of zinc sulfate, zinc gluconate, or zinc methionine. Dogs that absorb zinc poorly from the gastrointestinal tract must be given zinc intravenously. I recently completed a laboratory trial that demonstrated that a dietary enzyme supplement (Prozyme™) increased the absorption of zinc from the diet by over 30%.

Generic Dog Food Disease

Generic dog food disease was a condition recognized some years ago in dogs being fed generic (no name) dog foods. It is currently believed that some generic dog foods may contain ingredients that cause a relative zinc imbalance. This is assumed because the condition closely resembles zinc-responsive dermatosis, biopsies are consistent with those taken from dogs with that condition, and the animals completely recover when fed a regular dog food even though the generic dog food does contain adequate amounts of zinc according to the minimums suggested by the National Research Council (NRC). Affected animals are often healthy but covered by crusts.

Vitamin A-Responsive Dermatosis

Vitamin A-responsive dermatosis is also not a deficiency syndrome, but rather a skin condition that responds to high doses of vitamin A supplementation. The principal breed affected is the Cocker Spaniel, but other breeds (e.g., Labrador Retriever, Cairn Terrier) have also been reported with the condition. The syndrome is characterized by dandruff, hair loss, and marked crusting, especially bad on the back. The center of the problem is the hair follicle, where the scaling and crusting (follicular keratosis) begins. Diagnosis is confirmed by biopsies, and treatment includes megadoses of vitamin A daily, usually for life. The administration of high doses of vitamin A should not be taken lightly, since it can be toxic.

Fatty Acid Deficiency

Fatty acid deficiency is relatively rare, and only seen in dogs fed diets in which the fat content is deficient or not adequately preserved. Poor quality dog foods may be deficient in fatty acids. Dry foods especially are limited in the amount of fats that can be incorporated without going rancid. Antioxidants are normally added to foods to delay this process, but foods stored for a long time, especially at high temperatures, can lose their fatty acid content. Medical conditions that limit the ability of the body to absorb or metabolize ingested fats can also result in signs of fatty acid deficiency. These include chronic pancreatitis, liver disease, gall bladder disease, and malabsorption syndromes.

Animals must normally be on a fatty acid deficient diet for many months before they begin to show symptoms. A dry, lusterless coat and prominent dandruff are often the first effects noticed, followed by bacterial infections. Therapy involves feeding a good quality food with adequate fat content and supplementing the diet with a suitable fatty acid compound if necessary. Routine supplementation with fats is not recommended, and caution should be exercised in animals with pancreatitis, gall bladder disease, malabsorption syndromes, etc., where the increased fat in the diet can have medical consequences. Excessively high levels of fatty acids can actually interfere with the utilization of vitamin E. Topical applications of essential fatty acids will also result in some absorption, directly through the skin. Antiseborrheic shampoos will remove the scales and oiliness from the skin that often accompany this condition.

Vitamin E-Related Dermatosis

Vitamin E-related dermatosis has only been observed experimentally. It causes dryness of the skin and increased susceptibility to infection, scaling, and visual defects. It is very unlikely that many dogs suffer from vitamin E deficiency, although vitamin E has been used in the treatment of several disorders, including discoid and systemic lupus erythematosus, acanthosis nigricans, demodicosis, and epidermolysis bullosa simplex (dermatomyositis).

Dalmatian Bronzing Syndrome

Dalmatian bronzing syndrome is covered more completely in the chapter on breed-related skin problems. It results from an inability to handle certain proteins (purines) in the diet. These dogs have defects in their metabolism of uric acid, and when regular foods are fed, these dogs develop urinary tract problems, a coat that looks motheaten, scaling, and often a change in their coat color to a bronze hue. The exact reason for this color change has not been determined, but the condition can easily be controlled by limiting the amount of protein (especially purines) in the diet and/or by treating the dog with compounds that lower the blood uric acid levels. These diets can be purchased commercially (e.g., Hill's u/d) or formulated at home according to established recipes.

METABOLIC DERMATOSIS

A number of medical conditions have been associated with ill-defined dermatoses over the past few years. Under the general heading of metabolic dermatosis, these have been referred to by such terms as superficial necrolytic dermatitis, diabetic dermatopathy, hepatic dermatopathy, hepatocutaneous syndrome, glucagonoma syndrome, and necrolytic migratory erythema. These labels imply that there is some internal disease that is causing aberrations on the skin surface. Diabetes mellitus, liver/gall bladder disease, kidney disease, pancreatic disease, cancer, and defects of bile acid and uric acid metabolism have all been implicated. Since metabolic dermatosis was first reported in 1986, it has been the subject of intense scrutiny, and clearly the story is not yet complete.

This condition is recognized most often in older dogs (average age of 10 years), and most have some peculiar symptoms. Early on, affected dogs often have sores and blisters, which later become scaly and crusted. These are seen primarily on the feet, face, ears, genitals, and groin. In time many animals lose weight and may drink more and urinate more if they develop diabetes.

Diagnosis can be made on the basis of biopsy, but several other laboratory tests are needed in these dogs. Affected dogs usually have evidence of liver disease, high levels of glucagon (a hormone with effects opposite to insulin), glucose intolerance, and low blood levels of albumin, an important protein in the blood. X-ray and ultrasound examinations of the abdomen may be very helpful for identifying internal problems. It is suspected that the liver disease comes first, actually making these animals more susceptible to developing diabetes later, so if these dogs are tested early in the disease process, their blood sugar levels may not yet be abnormal.

Treatment for these animals is very difficult, since there is something very wrong in their metabolic makeup. Surgery may cure dogs with glucagon-secreting pancreatic tumors, but for the rest, the prognosis is quite poor. The average survival time is only a few months. In people, intensive treatment with certain amino acids may be helpful, but this research in dogs is still in its infancy.

SEBACEOUS ADENITIS

Periappendageal dermatitis (sebaceous adenitis) is becoming more and more common in dogs and is covered in more detail in the chapter on breed-related skin problems. Since it was originally reported in the Standard Poodle, it has now been recognized in many other breeds: Irish Setter, Collie, Samoyed, Miniature Poodle, Golden Retriever, Vizsla, Doberman Pinscher, Springer Spaniel, Basset Hound, Old English Sheepdog, Scottish Terrier, Akita, German Shepherd Dog, Miniature Pinscher, Chow Chow, Dachshund, Weimaraner, Lhasa Apso, Dalmatian, and even in mixed breeds.

The condition is named sebaceous adenitis because it appears that there is an inflammatory reaction in the sebaceous glands, the sebum-producing glands, that destroys them. Eventually, the skin in these areas becomes dry, scaly, and loses its hair. Diagnosis is made by biopsy. Strangely enough, sebaceous adenitis is neither painful nor itchy. Dogs that have it are in no distress and are not ill. Since the body does not replace sebaceous glands if they are completely destroyed, once this has occurred, the damage is permanent.

If these cases are diagnosed early enough, treatment is directed at curbing the inflammation. This may involve synthetic vitamin A derivatives and anti-inflammatory agents. Cyclosporine, the drug used in organ transplants, has also been used and has occasionally been helpful. Various topical products are used to condition the skin and keep it soft and hydrated. This is a lifelong project, but affected dogs continue to live a full, normal, and happy lifetime. They should not be used for breeding.

SCHNAUZER COMEDO SYNDROME

Schnauzer comedo syndrome (known as Schnauzer crud by breeders) is a familial disorder of Schnauzers in which keratin accumulates in the hair follicles and results in blackheads (comedones). It is most commonly found along the topline, where small bumps and scabs (crusts) appear. If these areas get infected, they may become quite itchy, and sometimes painful. The diagnosis can be confirmed by biopsy, but the clinical appearance is usually quite suggestive. Since approximately 25% of affected Schnauzers may also be hypothyroid, evaluation of thyroid function is also worthwhile.

Treatment is intensive, but affected dogs are usually in no real discomfort. If they have managed to acquire an infection, antibiotics will speed recovery. Hypothyroid dogs should be placed on appropriate supplementation. To cleanse the skin of comedones, frequent bathing is necessary, especially using benzoyl peroxide products or others that extend into the follicles. Alcohol wipes are often sufficient on small areas. Animals that are severely affected may need isotretinoin, a synthetic vitamin A derivative used for the management of acne in people.

FOLLICULAR DYSPLASIA

The term follicular dysplasia refers to a collection of disorders in which hair follicles that are normal at birth later become abnormal and nonfunctional, causing hair loss. In addition to the hair loss, the skin also often becomes dry and scaly. The condition is first seen most commonly in animals less than a year old.

There are several types of follicular dysplasia, some with similarities to the conditions that are described as color mutant alopecia, "gilding syndrome," black hair follicular dysplasia, and follicular dysplasia of Siberian Huskies.

There are no blood tests to confirm the diagnosis, and hormonal tests are invariably normal. Biopsies are needed to show the stage of growth of the follicles and any abnormalities they may have. While there is no cure for follicular dysplasia and animals that have it should not be used for breeding, the overall health of these dogs is not affected. Symptomatic therapy consists of lifelong antiseborrheic shampooing and often the use of emollient rinses, humectants, and moisturizers. Follicular dysplasia is covered in more detail in the chapter on breed-related skin problems.

CALLUS

Calluses are scaly or crusty pads that develop over pressure points subjected to repeated trauma. In time they become thickened, and invariably they get infected. Callus pyoderma is discussed in the chapter on bacterial and fungal skin problems. Calluses are most commonly seen on the elbows and hocks of large breeds of dogs, and occasionally on the sternum of others (e.g., Dachshunds). They are formed by the repeated impact of these body parts on hard surfaces, such as concrete, wood, or tile. The diagnosis is not difficult, but biopsies will eliminate any doubt.

For minor calluses, keeping animals off hard surfaces and applying moisturizers to the area is usually the only treatment required. For callus pyoderma, the use of antibiotics will also be necessary. Surgical removal of calluses is usually not a good idea—it can cause more problems than it corrects. For large calluses, protective pads (e.g., hockey elbow pads) will shield the areas from further trauma.

KERATOSES

Keratoses are accumulations of keratin on the skin surface and are discussed in more detail in the chapter on skin tumors. They can be further classified as seborrheic, lichenoid, actinic, or proliferative. The later two are the most important. Actinic keratoses are important because they reflect ultraviolet damage of the skin by sunlight and can evolve into sun-related cancers. Steps should be taken to protect the dog from further exposure to sun. Proliferative keratoses (cutaneous horns) are important because they tend to cover up underlying problems such as viral infections, cancers, and other keratoses. Additional tests should be run. The diagnosis can be confirmed by biopsy, and surgical removal usually cures the keratosis, but not necessarily the underlying problem.

LICHENOID DERMATOSES

Lichenoid dermatoses are named either for a distinctive clinical appearance or for a specific inflammatory pattern seen on biopsies. Clinically, lichenoid refers to a dense grouping of little bumps. On biopsy sections, lichenoid means that inflammatory cells are lining up and forming a dense band at the junction between the epidermis and the dermis. Clinical lichenoid dermatoses are uncommon in dogs and include idiopathic lichenoid dermatosis, lichenoid keratosis, and lichenoid-psoriasiform dermatitis of Springer Spaniels. Lichenoid biopsy findings have been associated with lupus erythematosus, pemphigus, pemphigoid, erythema multiforme, cutaneous T-cell-like lymphoma, uveodermatologic syndrome (Vogt-Koyanagi-Harada-like syndrome), toxic epidermal necrolysis, contact dermatitis, cheyletiellosis, lichenoid keratosis, lichenoid-psoriasiform dermatitis, and idiopathic lichenoid dermatitis.

Lichenoid-psoriasiform dermatitis of Springer Spaniels is probably hereditary. The dermatitis usually is manifested as bumps or wart-like or cauliflower-like projections of the ear flaps and sometimes the abdominal area, but sometimes they are all over the dog. Affected dogs are often less than three years old. The condition is more of a cosmetic defect than a health concern. Treatment with corticosteroids, antibiotics, or vitamin A does not alter the course of the disease, which waxes and wanes. Topical use of vitamin A derivatives may offer some benefit, but treatment should not be overdone, since the condition does not affect the health of these otherwise normal dogs.

6

IMMUNE-MEDIATED SKIN DISEASES

AUTOIMMUNE SKIN DISEASES

Although many different types of skin problems can be caused by an abnormally functioning immune system, the autoimmune skin diseases appear to be of special interest to both breeders and veterinarians. Autoimmune diseases are sometimes described in simplified terms as an allergy to oneself, but this is not the most accurate description of the condition. Allergies may result in nothing more serious than inflammation, while autoimmune diseases can actually destroy tissues. Neither are autoimmune diseases related to cancers; in autoimmune diseases abnormal antibodies are made by normal cells, not cancerous cells. Finally, autoimmune diseases are not like AIDS. The acquired immune deficiency virus causes an underactivity of the immune system; autoimmune diseases are the result of an overactive immune system.

Autoimmune skin diseases, therefore, result when an overactive immune system deposits abnormal antibodies in the skin, causing damage. Antibodies are supposed to act in a seek-and-destroy fashion, but they should be aimed at viruses, bacteria, and other intruders. In normal circumstances the body recognizes its own tissues and organs as "self" and leaves them alone. When the body recognizes something as foreign ("nonself"), the immune system reacts defensively to eliminate the foreign invader. This is what happens following transplant surgeries; the body recognizes the new tissue as foreign and tries to get rid of it, or "reject" it. In certain circumstances, however, the body may flex its immunological muscle and direct its defenses against one or many of its own tissues, producing autoantibodies. The result is an autoimmune disease.

Although much attention and interest is focused on autoimmune diseases, their significance must be kept in perspective, for they are relatively rare. For example, an average-sized veterinary hospital would be expected to encounter less than a dozen autoimmune skin diseases over the course of an entire year. The number seen by dermatologists is much higher, because they see referrals from hospitals in a wide geographic area.

Lupus Erythematosus

Lupus erythematosus (LE) is a disease that has been long recognized in animals and people and is characterized by the presence of many different autoantibodies that circulate in the blood and become deposited in a variety of tissues. Two forms have been recognized in animals, systemic lupus erythematosus and cutaneous (discoid) lupus erythematosus.

Systemic lupus erythematosus (SLE) is called "systemic" because it always involves more than one body system. It is also often missed as a diagnosis initially because it mimics so many other diseases. The most frequent clinical findings with SLE are fever that does not improve with antibiotics, arthritis, kidney disease, anemia, and skin problems, although many other disorders can arise. Collies, Shetland Sheepdogs, and perhaps Doberman Pinschers are the breeds most commonly affected.

Specific diagnostic testing for SLE includes a variety of blood tests and biopsies; confirmation is not always a simple matter. In people, the American Rheumatism Association has proposed a set of criteria that must be met before a diagnosis of SLE can be made, and some modified lists have been suggested for dogs. The important point is that a diagnosis cannot be accurately made on the basis of a suggestive rash, a single blood test, a single biopsy, or a set of symptoms.

In general, the minimum workup should include basic blood and urine tests, biopsies for histopathology, and an antinuclear antibody test (ANA). The basic blood tests are run to make sure that everything is functioning normally inside—after all, it's not called "systemic" lupus for nothing. The most common findings might include low red cell counts (anemia) and/or kidney problems. Biopsies are often taken from inflamed patches of skin, and sometimes special tests are also run on these samples to see if actual antibodies can be detected (immunopathology). The ANA is an important screening test for SLE in that it is frequently positive, but this test alone cannot confirm a diagnosis. It is not positive about 25% of the time in confirmed cases and may occasionally be positive in diseases that have nothing to do with SLE.

The therapy for SLE must be individualized but may be attempted with cortisone-like products (corticosteroids) and/or other medications that suppress the immune system and the production of abnormal antibodies. Therefore, therapies usually include prednisone, azathioprine (Imuran), and/or cyclophosphamide. Prednisone is the most common oral corticosteroid used; the others are treatments originally used for cancers and transplant patients. Unfortunately, all of these medications have potential side effects, so monitoring of blood and urine samples is an important part of the treatment program. Dogs must also be protected from sunlight, since, although it doesn't cause them, ultraviolet light makes any skin rashes worse and makes scarring more likely. Lupus is a scarring disease, and wherever the skin heals by scarring, hair cannot be expected to regrow.

Cutaneous (discoid) lupus erythematosus (CLE or DLE) is generally regarded as a less harmful form of SLE that doesn't involve tissues inside the body. It is most commonly seen as a rash on the face, but other areas may be involved as well. One of the most characteristic changes is a loss of pigment of the top of the nose and inside the nostrils. Collies, Shetland Sheepdogs, and Alaskan Malamutes appear to be most commonly affected, and many of the cases mistakenly labeled "Collie nose" are actually cutaneous lupus erythematosus. The important distinctions between systemic and cutaneous lupus erythematosus are that cutaneous lupus does not involve other body systems and that the vast majority of cases of cutaneous lupus never evolve into systemic lupus erythematosus. Of all the autoimmune skin diseases, cutaneous lupus does the least damage.

The diagnosis of cutaneous lupus erythematosus is not difficult, but often a full workup is done to be sure that you're not dealing with an early case of systemic lupus erythematosus that has no other symptoms yet.

The treatment of CLE/DLE differs from that of SLE in that heavy drug doses are usually not necessary. With CLE only the skin is involved, and therefore, in most cases, drugs capable of suppressing the entire immune system are not warranted. It is important that dogs with CLE not be "over-treated." Often, the use of immune-suppressing drugs in large doses is more of a health risk than the condition itself. Recently, the combination of an antibiotic (tetracycline) with a B vitamin (niacinamide) has been shown to be helpful in the management of cutaneous lupus. So at present, the best course of action in treating CLE is to limit sun exposure, use vitamin E to help lessen scarring, and consider using a niacinamide/tetracycline combination or relatively lower doses of corticosteroids. This may not achieve 100% control, but it will lessen the impact of the disease and allow the dog to live a relatively healthy, normal lifespan.

There are many differences between systemic and cutaneous lupus erythematosus when it comes to leading a normal life. Dogs with the cutaneous form of the disease can be expected to live a long and relatively normal life if cared for properly and if treatment is not excessive. On the other hand, dogs with systemic lupus must be treated aggressively and constantly monitored to be sure that other organs do not become involved. Both the disease and the treatments used to control it take their toll on dogs and humans alike and usually shorten their lifespans.

Pemphigus

The term pemphigus (Greek for blister) is used to describe four related but different blistering diseases, although blisters are rarely a prominent feature of the condition in dogs. The disease was named for the condition as it occurs in people, who develop blisters because their epidermis is relatively thick; the thinner epidermis of dogs means that these blisters quickly rupture or change into pustules (pimples).

There are currently four variants of pemphigus recognized in animals. Pemphigus vulgaris (PV) was first described in 1975, pemphigus foliaceus (PF) and pemphigus vegetans (PVe) in 1977, and pemphigus erythematosus (PE) in 1980. Pemphigus vulgaris is often the most aggressive form, followed by pemphigus foliaceus, pemphigus vegetans, and pemphigus erythematosus.

Pemphigus vulgaris is more an ulcerating disease than a blistering disease and tends to concentrate on regions where skin meets mucous membrane, such as the mouth, nose, lining of the eyes, rectum, vagina, nailbeds, and prepuce. Mouth problems are seen first in about 60% of cases, and eventually 90% of all dogs with pemphigus vulgaris have mouth problems involving the tongue, palate, or gums. Other favored areas include the armpits, groin area, footpads, and eyelids. This is a particularly severe disorder, but unlike systemic lupus erythematosus, internal organs remain unaffected.

Pemphigus vegetans is a very rare form of pemphigus that is believed to be a less harmful variation of pemphigus vulgaris. In this form, there are warty growths that become covered with pimples and often ooze fluid.

Pemphigus foliaceus is probably the most common form of pemphigus and also doesn't involve much blistering. In fact, pemphigus foliaceus is most often seen as a scaling rash that starts on the dog's face and head before becoming generalized. The mouth and mucous membranes are not usually involved in this disorder, but it is not unusual for the footpads to become thickened and scaly. When blisters do occur, they quickly evolve into pus-filled pimples and often resemble bacterial infections.

Pemphigus erythematosus is a less harmful variant of pemphigus folia-ceus and is, for the most part, limited to the face and head. Because it causes a facial rash, it is very similar to cutaneous lupus erythematosus. In fact, it was named pemphigus erythematosus because it was originally thought to be a combination or crossover of lupus erythematosus and pemphigus.

Even though the variants of pemphigus are quite different, the approach to diagnosis is similar for all. Because pemphigus is only "skin deep" and doesn't affect anything internally, routine blood tests should be normal. Specialized blood tests to detect circulating pemphigus autoantibodies are useful in people but have never been as helpful in dogs. One quick test that is helpful occasionally is the impression smear. To do this, a pimple or blister is "pricked," and the material is applied to a microscope slide and studied. If neither pimples nor blisters are available, the material found under a scab (crust) might provide a clue. The diagnosis is usually confirmed by biopsy findings if appropriate samples can be collected. What needs to be seen on the biposy is a blister, and since blisters are phenomenally short-lived in dogs, lasting perhaps two hours, the selection of appropriate biopsy sites is the most critical aspect of diagnosis. Occasionally, additional biopsies are also taken for immunologic tests such as direct immunofluorescent testing or immunoperoxidase testing. These tests performed on biopsy samples try to locate antibodies within the epidermis of the skin in a pattern characteristic of pemphigus. The tests are helpful when positive, but regular biopsies are still the most likely to actually provide a diagnosis.

The treatment of all forms of pemphigus is also similar, but it differs in degrees depending on the particular variant involved, the individual susceptibility, and the initial response to therapy. Prednisone remains the preferred first treatment, because it starts to work quickly, is inexpensive, and it's readily available. Unfortunately, corticosteroids alone are unsatisfactory in the majority of cases either because of side effects or because they are not completely effective, but better results can be achieved by combining them with other therapeutic agents such as azathioprine, chlorambucil, cyclophosphamide, or gold. Gold salt therapy (chrysotherapy), although it sounds exotic, is actually a very promising therapy for pemphigus and is not as expensive as one would imagine. Both injectable and oral forms are available, but most work in animals to date has used injectable gold salts. It is used together with corticosteroids such as prednisone because it takes so long to start working and because the side effects of the two drugs are not additive. Thus, corticosteroids coupled with either azathioprine or gold represents the best long-term choice in the treatment of pemphigus.

Pemphigoid

Pemphigoid (Greek for pemphigus-like) refers to a complex of blistering conditions similar to pemphigus, but in these the blister occurs deeper in the skin. Two types are known to occur in dogs, bullous pemphigoid and cicatricial pemphigoid.

In bullous pemphigoid (BP) the blisters are more apparent than in pemphigus because of their deeper location, beneath the epidermis. Collies, Shetland Sheepdogs, and perhaps Doberman Pinschers appear to be most often affected. Clinically, bullous pemphigoid appears similar to pemphigus vulgaris, and blisters, ulcers, and crusts may be seen in the mouth, nose, face, armpits, and groin. Although animals may have a fever and seem sick with bullous pemphigoid, there is no internal spread of the disease.

Similar to pemphigus, the only way to reliably diagnose bullous pemphigoid is to get appropriate biopsy samples. Occasionaly biopsies are taken for specialized immunologic tests (direct immunofluorescence or immunoperoxidase), but these only occasionally provide more information than the standard biopsies. The most important aspect of diagnosis is to send the biopsies to pathologists with special expertise in diseases of the skin. Blood tests, which are often helpful in diagnosing people with bullous pemphigoid, do not work well in dogs.

The treatment of bullous pemphigoid is identical to that of pemphigus vulgaris. Drugs that suppress the immune system are used to force down the level of abnormal antibodies so they cannot cause problems. Prednisone is often used initially, but often other medications are needed for long-term maintenance. The most common drugs used for control are azathioprine, cyclophosphamide, and gold salts. Because all of these medications have side effects, periodic monitoring is an important aspect of long-term control.

Cicatricial, or mucous membrane pemphigoid, is a chronic blistering disease affecting primarily the mouth and eyelids. It differs from bullous pemphigoid only in that the problems remain localized rather than spreading to other parts of the body. Biopsies cannot distinguish between bullous and cicatricial pemphigoid; this distinction is made on the basis of clinical signs and the extent of disease.

Because the affected areas are localized, cicatricial pemphigoid is simpler to treat than bullous pemphigoid. Occasionally the problem can be controlled with topical therapy alone; both corticosteroids and cyclosporine A have been successfully used for this purpose.

Uveodermatological (Vogt-Koyanagi-Harada-like) Syndrome

Uveodermatological syndrome, also known as Vogt-Koyanagi-Harada-like (VKH) syndrome after the individuals who described the syndrome in man, is believed to be an autoimmune disease leveled against melanocytes, the cells responsible for producing pigment. Since these cells are found in the skin, eyes, and surface of the brain, problems can arise at any of these locations. Individually, the eye problem is referred to as granulomatous panuveitis, pigment loss of the hair as poliosis, and pigment loss of the skin as vitiligo. Unlike people, dogs rarely have deafness, meningitis, or other neurological symptoms associated with this disorder.

Granulomatous panuveitis is a severe eye disorder that can result in blindness if not recognized and treated promptly. Since the onset of symptoms can be quite rapid, veterinary evaluation should not be postponed. Skin changes include loss of pigment of the nose, lips, eyelids, and occasionally the entire body. Most affected dogs are in young adulthood (1–6 years of age), and the Akita appears to be the breed affected most often. Other breeds at increased risk include the Irish Setter, Siberian Husky, Samoyed, Shetland Sheepdog, and Chow Chow. The acute blindness that accompanies the syndrome is usually more alarming than the loss of pigment.

The diagnosis of VKH relies on appropriate biopsies. The mainstay of therapy is topical and/or systemic corticosteroids. Chemotherapeutic drugs such as azathioprine and cyclophosphamide have also been helpful in treatment. Once blindness has occurred, the return of sight is unlikely, but early therapeutic intervention is usually successful.

Alopecia Areata

Alopecia areata means "an area of hair loss." The condition is presumed to be due to an immune-mediated attack on growing hair follicles. This is most often seen as a patch of hair loss on smooth skin that doesn't seem to be inflamed. In people, there is at least circumstantial evidence that the disorder is autoimmune in nature, and this theory has been extended to dogs (rightly or wrongly). Actually, alopecia areata is not a dangerous disorder at all and it really represents a patch of baldness with no health risks.

The diagnosis can be confirmed by biopsy if the samples are sent to a pathologist with expertise in disorders of the skin. The biopsies show a collection of white blood cells (lymphocytes) preying on growing hair follicles. Once the hair follicle goes into a resting stage, any inflammation that might have occurred subsides. This leaves a patch of smooth skin without hair. Biopsies are important, because other diseases (e.g., ringworm, bacteria, rabies vaccination sites) may look quite similar yet are treated quite differently. Interestingly enough, after the inflammation has subsided, the lack of growing hair follicles is very similar to conditions produced by hormonal disorders such as hypothyroidism, and this mistaken diagnosis may be made if the pathologist is not provided with accurate clinical information.

For the most part, alopecia areata is not treated, since it really doesn't affect the health of a dog. Since increasing the blood supply to the hairless patch of skin may cause the follicles to go back into a growth phase, using a mildly abrasive brushing technique (for many weeks or months) may stimulate the hair to grow in affected areas. Injections of corticosteroids may also cause hair to grow, but treatment must not be excessive or the side effects may be more troublesome than the disease itself. Minoxidil (Rogaine), used in the treatment of male pattern baldness, has also been used for alopecia areata but is not licensed for treatment of dogs.

Eosinophilic Granuloma

Canine eosinophilic granuloma appears to be an immune-mediated disorder, most commonly affecting Siberian Huskies. Most of these affected dogs are male and young, usually less than 3 years old.

Although dogs may have associated lumps on their flanks and underside, most dogs with eosinophilic granuloma are healthy but develop nodules in their mouth. These nodules are raised and red and may be confused with tumors.

The diagnosis is made by biopsy. The findings are very similar to linear granuloma in the cat and Well's syndrome in humans. Unfortunately, the causes of these conditions are not well understood either.

Treatment is based on suppressing the immune system, and the condition is quite responsive to corticosteroids, often at doses much less than needed to control the other autoimmune diseases. Sometimes eosinophilic granuloma improves spontaneously, even without treatment.

OTHER IMMUNE-MEDIATED SKIN DISEASES

Erythema Multiforme

Erythema multiforme is an immune reaction of the body to a variety of potential offenders. In people, the most common initiators are recurrent *Herpes simplex* or mycoplasmal infection and drug reactions. The name itself means "redness of the skin appearing in many different forms."

Although somewhat arbitrarily, very severe forms of erythema multiforme are often referred to as erythema multiforme major or sometimes toxic epidermal necrolysis (TEN). Most erythema multiforme is limited to the skin, but toxic epidermal necrolysis is as devastating as a second degree burn and can result in fever, shock, and even death.

Since erythema multiforme in dogs most often represents a reaction to bacterial infections or to drugs, drug exposure must be carefully evaluated in suspected cases. Biopsies are often needed to help confirm the diagnosis, but they do not detect the underlying cause. Uncovering that may involve some medical detective work. If the problem is identified and corrected, the erythema multiforme typically resolves, on its own, in 3–6 weeks. TEN is potentially life-threatening and requires intravenous fluid therapy.

Cutaneous Vasculitis

Cutaneous vasculitis is a name given to a collection of disorders that cause damage to blood vessels in the skin. If immune complexes (collections of antibodies and their targets) get caught up in the small blood vessels of the skin, they can severely damage those vessels and result in the death of the skin (necrosis) nourished by those vessels. While problems can occur anywhere in the body, they are most frequent on the extremities, the feet and ears.

In these areas, blotches (petechiae) may be seen, or there may be an elevated bruise (purpura), or there may be actual notching of the skin (necrosis), especially on the ears. This "ear notching" is most commonly seen in Dachshunds, so there may be a genetic component to vasculitis in this breed.

When it comes to identifying the cause of the vasculitis, there are many possibilities to be considered, including a variety of infections, drug reactions, other immune-mediated diseases (e.g., lupus), bug bites, chronic diseases (e.g., diabetes mellitus), or even exposure to cold (cold agglutinin disease).

Because so many different underlying problems can result in vasculitis, diagnostic testing can get quite involved. The diagnosis can be confirmed by biopsy, but several different tests (e.g., ANA, circulating immune complexes, microbial cultures, tests for infectious diseases) may be needed to identify the true underlying cause.

As it is with many other skin disorders, the treatment of vasculitis is most successful if directed against the true cause of the problem. If this cannot be identified, symptomatic control is usually instituted with corticosteroids. Several sulfa-based drugs, such as dapsone and sulfasalazine, are often used when corticosteroids don't work well enough, but these have potential side effects of their own.

Nodular Panniculitis

Nodular panniculitis is not strictly an immune-mediated disorder. It reflects damage to the fat beneath the skin, the panniculus. Anything that interferes with the blood supply to the fat will result in damage, and although infections and even pancreatitis are sometimes implicated, most insults are caused by the immune system. Since damage to the fat results in an inflamed lump, this condition is frequently mistaken for a cancer, which it is not.

Juvenile panniculitis is seen in dogs under 6 months of age, although similar syndromes have been reported in older dogs. The most commonly affected breeds are Dachshunds, Toy Poodles, Collies, and Wirehaired Fox Terriers. The disorder is seen as relatively painless lumps usually confined to the neck, trunk, and legs. The nodules can rupture and discharge an oily material or can spontaneously dry up and leave depressed scars. The diagnosis is made by biopsy, and a short course (about two weeks) of corticosteroids is usually enough to cure the problem.

Other immune causes of nodular panniculitis include lupus erythematosus, dermatomyositis, scleroderma, and erythema nodosum. These tend to cause a panniculitis that is more chronic and more difficult to treat. Biopsy findings are critical, as are routine blood profiles, ANA tests, and microbial cultures. Treatment needs to be directed against the underlying cause.

Nonimmunologic causes of nodular panniculitis are many, including infections, cysts, cancer, reactions to injections, and trauma to the area. Also, in some dogs with pancreatic disease, the enzymes released can cause digestion of fat, which can result in panniculitis. An interesting form of panniculitis that has been reported recently is a reaction to rabies vaccination, and although several breeds appear predisposed, the Miniature Poodle has accounted for the most cases to date. The cause is still being investigated, but some dogs develop a reaction when the vaccine is administered into the fat; several weeks or even months after vaccination, the dog may develop a round, smooth, hairless patch. The hairless area is painless and there are no health complications, but hair is unlikely to regrow in that spot.

Scleroderma

Scleroderma is an immunologic disease that causes the skin to become thickened and firm. Although there is a systemic, potentially fatal variant in people, only the localized form (morphea) has been reported in dogs. Affected dogs have patches of smooth but thickened skin, which, for the most part, has lost the hair.

The diagnosis is made by biopsy, and since this is such a rare disease in dogs, pathologists with expertise in skin are the only ones likely to recognize the inflammatory pattern. The localized form in dogs is relatively benign, and treatment is not always needed. When treatment is warranted, localized injections of corticosteroids are often selected.

Sjögren's Syndrome

Sjögren's syndrome is more of an eye disorder than a skin disease, but it is actually a "dryness complex" of dry eyes (keratoconjunctivitis sicca), dry mouth (xerostomia), and a connective tissue component such as lupus erythematosus or rheumatoid arthritis. Affected dogs frequently have patches of dry skin, often with dandruff.

The diagnosis is best made by biopsying the lacrimal (tear) glands rather than the skin. In addition, about 42% of affected dogs have a positive ANA test, and 34% are positive for rheumatoid factor.

Treatment is often attempted initially with corticosteroids, but some recent work with cyclosporine A has been very encouraging.

Juvenile Cellulitis

Juvenile cellulitis, also referred to as puppy strangles, is an immune-mediated inflammatory disease most commonly seen in young Dachshunds, Golden Retrievers, and Pointers. Originally it was thought to be a bacterial disease and was treated with a wide variety of antibiotics, but this therapy never seemed to be totally effective.

It is now believed that these young pups, for some reason, develop a transient immune-mediated disease that can be effectively "cured" by as little as two weeks of drug therapy. These pups often develop severely swollen faces, and the lymph nodes in the throat area become enlarged and corded. Diagnosis should be made on the basis of biopsies so that appropriate therapy can begin.

Unlike most other immune-mediated disorders, juvenile cellulitis usually clears completely with two weeks' worth of heavy-dose corticosteroids and almost never recurs. Pups recover as though they had never had the problem. It is important that these pups be monitored carefully throughout the course of therapy so the dosage can be adjusted if necessary and to guard against corticosteroid-induced side effects in these young animals.

Sterile Pyogranuloma

Sterile pyogranuloma is a perplexing, presumably immune-mediated disease that was originally thought to be a bacterial infection that occurred between the toes. It is one of the causes of interdigital dermatitis and is frequently misdiagnosed as "interdigital cysts." Great Danes, St. Bernards, Newfoundlands, Dachshunds, and English Bulldogs appear to get the disease most often.

It is easy to see how the condition could be mislabeled as "cysts," because nodules clearly form between the toes and often ooze blood, serum, or pus. It is thought that the disorder represents the deposit of abnormal antibodies between the toes, but this has been hard to prove. Because bacteria frequently are also involved, it is not unusual for biopsies to identify the problem as a severe bacterial infection even though it didn't start as one. Also, if bacterial cultures are taken from infected sites, it is not surprising that the laboratory tests will confirm the presence of bacteria. However, carefully collected samples from sites that have not yet opened to the surface will usually be sterile on culture, attesting to the fact that bacteria come in later and don't actually cause the problem.

Treatment is usually successful with corticosteroids or other drugs that suppress the body's immune response. Antibiotics will clear the surface infection, but if the underlying problem is not addressed, the infection will soon recur.

Sterile Eosinophilic Pustulosis

Sterile eosinophilic pustulosis is a rare problem in which itchy pimples develop for no apparent reason. In time, the skin can become darker in these regions and the hair can fall out.

Diagnosis is made by biopsy, but it is critical that more common causes such as allergies, bacterial infections, and parasites be carefully considered, because the biopsy findings in these are very similar. The condition gets its name because the pimples are infiltrated with eosinophils, a type of white blood cell associated with immunologic reactions and parasites, and microbes do not appear to be involved—hence "sterile."

Treatment is often with moderate doses of corticosteroids that may need to be maintained indefinitely. Relapses are common when treatment is discontinued.

Subcorneal Pustular Dermatosis

This is a rare skin problem that has been suggested to be immune-mediated in people, so we presume that the same is true in dogs. Miniature Schnauzers are the breed most commonly affected.

With this disorder, the general health remains unchanged, but crops of pimples come and go, affecting predominantly the trunk and head. The pimples quickly rupture and leave little scabs (crusts) and scale. The condition waxes and wanes on its own accord and doesn't seem to respond consistently to either antibiotics or corticosteroids.

Diagnosis is made by biopsy, and the findings are often similar to pemphigus foliaceus and superficial bacterial infections. It takes a well-trained pathologist with a special interest in skin problems to reliably make the distinction. Treatment is often instituted with dapsone, a drug related to the sulfas, and because of potential side effects, the dog must be carefully monitored.

Dermatitis Herpetiformis

Dermatitis herpetiformis is extremely rare in dogs and causes an itchy eruption primarily on the trunk, head, ears, and feet. It is associated with an intestinal problem, a gluten sensitivity, that causes a specific form of antibody (IgA) to be deposited in the skin.

Because this disorder is so phenomenally rare, cases should be confirmed by regular biopsies, direct immunofluorescence testing of biopsies, and by detecting IgA circulating immune complexes.

For actual cases of dermatitis herpetiformis, treatment usually consists of feeding a gluten-restricted diet and often treating with a sulfa-related drug, dapsone. Because of the potential side effects of dapsone, dogs should be regularly monitored with blood counts and liver function profiles.

IMMUNE DEFICIENCY SYNDROMES

Immune deficiency disorders have been recognized for years in dogs, but research to date is still scant. Deficiencies can be inherited or acquired and can involve any aspect of the immune system.

Immunoglobulin A Deficiency

Immunoglobulin A (IgA) deficiency is probably the most common immunoglobulin deficiency in dogs. It is most commonly reported in the Chinese Shar-pei, German Shepherd Dog, and Beagle. In one study, 70% of Chinese Shar-peis studied were found to be IgA deficient. IgA is a family of antibodies that protect the surface areas of the body (rather than internal organs), so deficiencies may result in recurrent infection of the skin, ears, respiratory tract, or digestive system. The diagnosis is made by measuring blood levels of IgA. The measurement is most accurate if a specimen from a normal dog of the same age can be sent to the laboratory for comparison purposes. Treatment is often with long-term antibiotics, since no specific therapies exist to stimulate production of IgA by the body. Nonspecific immune stimulants such as staphyloccocal bacterin and thymus gland extracts may be beneficial but have not been completely evaluated for this purpose. It is best if affected dogs can be kept away from other animals that may be harboring infection, and they should be subjected to as little stress as possible. Although some animals appear to outgrow their susceptibility to infection, this should not be anticipated.

Immunoincompetence

Incompetence of the immune system is probably quite common, but current testing makes it difficult to confirm this suspicion in most cases. Animals that have recurrent bacterial infections, demodicosis, or dermatophytosis probably have an immune system that is not functioning adequately. We suspect that the T-cell system or so-called cell-mediated/lymphokine-mediated response is where the problem lies; this is the same arm of the immune system that is disturbed in people with AIDS. But it does little good to modify the HIV test for dogs, because the AIDS virus does not affect dogs. The lymphocyte blastogenesis assay gives a very crude measure of the T-cell system, but it is available from only very few laboratories. Most of the time the diagnosis must be made without sufficient confirmation. When animals develop infections that we can't explain in any other fashion, we frequently suspect immunoincompetence but don't have the luxury of proving it. Treatment options are also somewhat limited. Initially, antibiotics are used to treat infections, but for long-term plans, immune stimulants are worthwhile options.

Canine Cyclic Hematopoiesis

Canine cyclic hematopoiesis, formerly called Gray Collie syndrome, has been reported in silver-gray Collies, Pomeranians, and Cocker Spaniels. It is covered in more detail in the chapter on breed-related skin problems. Animals have a defect in their neutrophils, a type of white blood cell, causing them to swing from high levels to low levels on a regular schedule. When white blood cell counts are at their lowest, these dogs are very prone to developing severe infections, diarrhea, painful joints, and, sometimes, hemorrhage. Most die during these episodes, and at a very young age.

Canine Granulocytopathy Syndrome

Canine granulocytopathy syndrome is a relatively rare inherited disorder seen in Irish Setters. These animals can produce neutrophils (a type of white blood cell) in adequate amounts, but these cells cannot do their job of killing bacteria. Affected dogs often suffer from severe infections, especially recurrent pyoderma and osteomyelitis, an infection of the bone marrow. The diagnosis can only be made by neutrophil function tests, which are only available from specialized laboratories.

A similar syndrome has been described in young Weimaraners, associated with neutrophil defects and immunoglobulin deficiencies. These dogs develop fever, vomiting, diarrhea, arthritis, bleeding tendencies, and a variety of other symptoms.

Combined Immunodeficiency

Combined immunodeficiency is a devastating inherited disease reported in Dachshunds and Basset Hounds. These dogs have a greatly impaired immune response and are susceptible to life-threatening viral, bacterial, and fungal diseases. Most die before they are a year old. Diagnosis can be made by performing specialized tests on lymphocytes, neutrophils, and immunoglobulins. No treatment is effective and most affected dogs die before they can be bred; parents and close relatives should not be used for breeding.

Thymus Gland Disorders

The thymus gland is very large in puppies and is an important regulator of immune function. The thymus programs the T-cells, special lymphocytes that patrol the body perimeter and keep it safe from invasion. When the thymus does not develop properly, "wasting syndromes" and recurrent infection can occur in pups. A number of nongenetic processes can adversely affect development of the thymus, including parvovirus infection and zinc deficiency. Some disorder of the thymus gland is also suspected to be involved with the lethal acrodermatitis syndrome seen in Bull Terriers. A similar condition has been reported in Weimaraners that have a growth hormone deficiency, a small thymus, and too few T-lymphocytes. They are prone to many different infections, and without appropriate therapy, will die within a few weeks or months. These pups have been shown to respond to supplementation with growth hormone or the thymic hormone thymosin fraction 5.

Unfortunately, it is currently very difficult to evaluate thymus function in the living animal. If pups die, the thymus is often examined, weighed, and biopsied to see if it was affected, but currently there are no blood tests for the thymic hormones thymosin, thymopoietin, thymic humoral factor, and thymulin. These hormones are also very expensive and not generally available to be used for treatment. Crude thymus gland extracts are available for use but have not yet been extensively studied.

7

ENDOCRINE (HORMONAL) SKIN PROBLEMS

The endocrine system is a complex collection of glands that produce hormones and secrete them directly into the bloodstream. Endocrine skin diseases actually reflect disorders of the thyroid gland, adrenal gland, pituitary gland, hypothalamus, thymus, and sex organs. All of these glands produce hormones of one kind or another that can cause skin problems in animals. Some diseases are caused when hormone levels get too low (e.g., hypothyroidism), some are caused when levels are too high (e.g., Cushing's disease), and others may be an indirect reflection of disease (e.g., growth hormone-responsive dermatosis).

For the most part, the endocrine organs work very much like the thermostat in a house. The body is constantly measuring the amount of different hormones in the bloodstream. Most of this information is actually processed in the hypothalamus and pituitary, which are located at the base of the brain. When a hormone gets above normal, the system shuts down for a while until the level drops; when hormones drop below a certain point, the system kicks in and starts producing more, and the levels rise once again. This is known as a negative-feedback mechanism.

This is a simplified version of the endocrine system, of course; the real system functions with a variety of different hormones, not just one. And because hormone levels in the blood fluctuate so widely throughout the day, taking one blood sample and hoping for a diagnosis is often wishful thinking. Very often it is necessary to "stimulate" the system or "suppress" it to see how high or low the levels actually go, or to perform more exacting tests. This often complicates the diagnostic process and makes it more expensive, but unfortunately, there are rarely easy answers.

The endocrine disorders with the most bearing on dermatology are hypothyroidism, hyperadrenocorticism, growth hormone-responsive dermatosis, and sex hormone disorders.

HYPOTHYROIDISM

Hypothyroidism is the most commonly diagnosed endocrine disorder in dogs. It describes a condition caused by a low level of thyroid hormones in the blood. As discussed above, thyroid hormones are produced as a joint venture of the hypothalamus, the pituitary gland, and the thyroid gland. It works this way: Thyrotropin-releasing hormone (TRH) is produced in the hypothalamus of the brain. This then stimulates the pituitary gland, located at the base of the brain, to secrete another hormone, thyroid-stimulating hormone (TSH). Finally, TSH stimulates the thyroid gland to produce two hormones, thyroxine (T-4) and triiodothyronine (T-3). Both of these hormones circulate in the blood tightly bound to proteins, but only once released do these "free" hormones actually exert any effect. Approximately 99% of the hormone is tightly bound to protein and not active and only about 1% of the hormone is in its "free" active form. The bound portion serves as a reservoir of hormone while the "free" portion actually does all the work. Thyroxine (T-4) is later converted to T-3 and reverse T-3 (rT-3), principally in the liver and kidneys. Although hypothyroidism may be due to low levels of either T-4 or T-3, clearly T-4 is the more important hormone and the one most likely to cause problems in hypothyroidism.

Why do dogs develop hypothyroidism? As it is in people, the most common cause of hypothyroidism in dogs is an immune-mediated process in which antibodies attack and destroy the thyroid gland. This is referred to most often as lymphocytic thyroiditis. In people, the disease is often called Hashimoto's thyroiditis. The second most common cause is idiopathic follicular atrophy, degeneration of the thyroid tissue for no apparent reason. And there is now much evidence that many cases of hypothyroidism have a genetic basis. A great many breeds are prone to developing hypothyroidism, including Afghan Hounds, Akitas, Alaskan Malamutes, Boxers, Brittany Spaniels, Chinese Shar-peis, Chow Chows, Cocker Spaniels, Dachshunds, Doberman Pinschers, English Bulldogs, Golden Retrievers, Great Danes, Irish Setters, Irish Wolfhounds, Newfoundlands, Pomeranians, Poodles, and

Schnauzers. Other breeds with suspected tendencies to hypothyroidism include Airedale Terriers, Australian Shepherds, Basset Hounds, Beagles, Bouviers des Flandres, Briards, Collies, Corgis, English Springer Spaniels, English Setters, German Shepherd Dogs, Gordon Setters, Irish Water Spaniels, Keeshonden, Kuvaszok, Labrador Retrievers, Mastiffs, Old English Sheepdogs, Samoyeds, Shetland Sheepdogs, Soft-coated Wheaton Terriers, Vizslas, and Weimaraners.

There are many misconceptions about the clinical signs (symptoms) of hypothyroidism and how it is best diagnosed. It is important to note that approximately one-third of hypothyroid dogs won't have any skin problems at all. Many people also want to reserve the diagnosis for dogs that are over-weight but obesity is only rarely associated with hypothyroidism. In fact, many dogs will be entirely normal until they have completely used up their reserve of thyroid hormone which may take several years.

The clinical signs exhibited by hypothyroid dogs are quite diverse. Approximately a third of hypothyroid dogs don't have any skin problems at all, but severely affected dogs may have one or more of the following characteristics: lethargy, recurrent bacterial infections, noninflammatory hair loss equally distributed along both sides of the back (bilaterally symmetric alopecia), dull, dry, lusterless haircoat, increased pigmentation of the skin, scaling and oiliness of the skin, a tendency toward obesity, inability to tolerate cold, and puffiness under the skin (myxedema). In the most extreme form of hypothyroidism, animals may become comatose.

When it comes to hypothyroidism, don't try to make a checklist of symptoms to match up with your canine. If conscientious care is being given, breeds at risk can be screened when they are completely without symptoms. Thyroiditis usually starts between one and three years of age and progresses throughout middle age and may only be clinically detectable later in life. In the meantime, the immune-mediated process may continue to make animals more susceptible to other immunologic diseases.

As animals lose thyroid reserve from ongoing destruction of thyroid tissue, an important dynamic takes place. When the available or "free" levels of T-4 start to drop, the body compensates by having the pituitary gland secrete more TSH which in turn results in more T-4 being produced by the diseased thyroid gland. Because the levels of T-4 in the blood are normal, these animals often appear symptom-free and this stops most from getting appropriate veterinary attention.

When it comes to diagnosing hypothyroidism, veterinarians usually rely on a variety of blood tests. Because of the complexity of the thyroid hormone system, the "best" test for thyroid function is the subject of much controversy. In all dogs suspected of having hypothyroidism, it is also worth submitting blood samples for routine hematologic and biochemical profiles. Over 50% of hypothyroid dogs have high blood cholesterol and often increased triglycerides and lipoproteins as well. A small percentage of affected dogs are also anemic.

A test measuring simply T-3 and T-4 levels is easy to perform and inexpensive but quite unreliable, since thyroid hormone levels fluctuate greatly throughout the day. There is thus a great interpretive problem, since at any one time, thyroid levels may be normal in 30–60% of hypothyroid dogs and abnormal in 20% of normal dogs. This will also not detect early cases in which the T-4 and T-3 levels would still be expected to be in normal range. There is also some variation in normal thyroid levels related to age, breed, and sex. Puppies have total thyroxine concentrations two to five times the normal adult concentrations until about 4 months of age. After that time, levels continuously decrease with age. There is also some breed variability and the Greyhound has been shown to have lower T-4 levels and higher T-3 levels than mixed-breed dogs. As a general rule (with exceptions), small-breed dogs have higher concentrations of T-4 than do larger breeds. Finally, concentrations of T-4 and T-3 are consistently higher in bitches that are pregnant or in diestrus.

Tests that measure free levels of T-4 and T-3 are now available from specialized laboratories and measure the small percentage of hormone not bound to protein and available to the tissues. Free levels are a much more sensitive indicator of hypothyroidism than the "total" levels that fluctuate greatly throughout the day.

The classic diagnostic test has been the TSH stimulation test, in which baseline blood T-4 and T-3 levels are determined. TSH is injected intravenously and a second blood sample is obtained in 4–8 hours. This measures the ability of the thyroid gland to respond to maximal stimulation and is a useful test, though TSH is expensive and difficult to obtain. Because of the difficulty in obtaining TSH, a TRH stimulation test is also possible and usually gives comparable results.

In people, measuring actual levels of TSH in the blood is very helpful, but to date, a reliable test measuring canine TSH is not available. One has been developed but preliminary studies have not been encouraging. Human test kits cannot reliably measure canine TSH and therefore have not proved useful. Continued research is bound to provide additional options.

Thyroid autoantibodies, the most common initiators of hypothyroidism, can now be measured by specialized laboratories but must be evaluated with caution. There appears to be a genetic predilection in Great Danes, Irish Setters, and Old English Sheepdogs for producing autoantibodies. In Borzoi dogs, lymphocytic thyroiditis has been shown to be an inherited trait. It is also important to note that high levels of autoantibody only indicate risk; they do not confirm a diagnosis. Only approximately 50% of hypothyroid dogs have these antibodies.

What is the best approach for owners with breeds at risk of becoming hypothyroid? At this point, it would seem prudent to perform a blood count, biochemical profile (including cholesterol), and a thyroid profile (total and free levels of T-4 and T-3) at 1 year of age and annually thereafter. For certain breeds, such as the Great Dane, Old English Sheepdog, and Irish Setter, it would also be advisable to measure thyroid hormone autoantibody levels. For breeds that are not at high risk, it would be advisable to measure baseline thyroid hormone levels at 5–7 years of age and annually thereafter.

Many dogs evaluated for thyroid function have values that aren't clearly hypothyroid and are often referred to as borderline cases. Remember, the levels of all hormones are in a constant state of flux and many things can interfere with a single measurement. Many drugs, especially corticosteroids, phenylbutazone, seizure medications and sulfas, profoundly influence the levels of thyroid hormones in circulation. Also, any problem that causes animals not to eat properly for more than two days can dramatically affect thyroid hormone levels. A number of diseases are known to affect thyroid hormone levels: diabetes mellitus, Cushing's disease, kidney disease, liver disease, congestive heart failure, and others. Sex hormones can also profoundly affect testing, so thyroid profiles are difficult to interpret in intact females within two months following estrus (heat). Although these "borderline" animals are typically put on a six-week trial course of thyroid supplementation, an interesting alternative is to measure the circulating levels of reverse T-3 in the blood, which is often increased when thyroid levels are decreased by processes other than thyroid disease.

Treatment

Even though the diagnosis of hypothyroidism may be somewhat complicated, treatment is easy and relatively inexpensive. It involves supplementing the hormone (T-4) that is lacking and doses can be calculated by body weight or by body surface area. Since T-3 in the body is created from T-4, it is not necessary to use T-3 supplements, which are typically quite expensive.

Treatment involves giving a prescribed dose of thyroid hormone twice daily, for life. Typically, patients are re-evaluated after six weeks on therapy and thyroid levels measured 4–6 hours after the morning pill was given. This represents the highest level the thyroid hormones are going to reach. If levels are well into normal range, once-daily dosing may be considered, but most dogs are maintained on twice-daily treatment for life. After this, levels should be repeated annually, to insure that the pet is still being maintained in normal range and that the dosage does not need to be altered. Skin problems associated with hypothyroidism usually resolve in two to three months.

HYPERADRENOCORTICISM (CUSHING'S DISEASE)

Hyperadrenocorticism is commonly referred to as Cushing's disease or Cushing's syndrome and describes a condition in which the body produces too much cortisol, its own form of cortisone. Cortisol is produced in the adrenal glands, which are located at the top poles of the kidneys.

The adrenals work on a negative feedback mechanism which relies on corticotropin-releasing factor (CRF) from the hypothalamus and adreno-corticotropic hormone (ACTH) from the pituitary gland. The way it works is this—when blood levels of cortisol get below normal, CRF is released from the hypothalamus which causes ACTH to be released from the pituitary which, in turn, causes the adrenals to release cortisol into the blood.

Abnormally high levels of cortisol can result from problems—usually tumors—in the brain (hypothalamus or pituitary) or in the adrenals them-selves. In addition, animals stressed by such chronic conditions as diabetes mellitus, liver disease, and kidney disease may have abnormal cortisol levels. Most tumors of the pituitary are benign but result in the secretion of ACTH which, in turn, causes high levels of cortisol. About half of the adrenal tumors are malignant and half benign. Various breeds are prone to hyperadrenocorti-cism, especially the Boxer, Boston Terrier, Poodle, and Dachshund.

When cortisone-like medications are given to treat medical conditions, they can cause side effects that mimic symptoms of the natural disease. This is referred to as iatrogenic Cushing's syndrome. It can result from the use of injectable corticosteroids, tablets, liquids, eye drops, creams, or ointments.

The symptoms of cortisol excess are quite variable, since some animals are more tolerant of changes in their blood cortisols than others. Therefore, some dogs show symptoms immediately, but others may seem normal for years. About two-thirds of cushingoid dogs will have increased thirst (poly-dipsia), increased urination (polyuria), and increased hunger (polyphagia) associated with their disease. These are some of the same side effects that are seen when dogs are given corticosteroids for medical treatment. Perhaps half of all dogs with Cushing's disease have hair loss equally distributed along both sides of the back (bilaterally symmetric alopecia) that is not associated with any inflammation. High blood pressure is seen in perhaps 60% of cases. Because cortisone interferes with the body's immune responses, it is not unusual for affected dogs to also be more susceptible to infection. Other clinical signs that might be seen include thinning of the skin, plugged hair follicles (blackheads) on the underside, muscle atrophy, an enlarged liver due to fatty deposits, and abnormal behavior. More bizarre symptoms may be evident if animals have large tumors associated with their disease pressing on surrounding organs, especially within the brain.

Hyperadrenocorticism may be suspected on the basis of the history, clinical signs, blood and urine test results, and skin biopsy, but confirma-tion requires measuring specific levels of the different hormones involved in this condition.

Since Cushing's disease is seen mostly in middle-aged to older dogs, suspi-cious findings may be evident when dogs are seen annually and given geriatric workups. Most geriatric evaluations are done annually, starting when dogs are about 7 years of age and include blood tests, urine tests, and radiographs (x-rays). Some findings that may be suggesting of Cushing's disease includ e recurrent urinary tract infections, high blood sugar, high cholesterol, and increased liver enzymes (serum alkaline phosphatase, serum alanine trans- aminase). Radiographs might reveal an enlarged liver, osteoporosis, abnormal calcium deposits in tissues or even calcified adrenal tumors.

Unfortunately, measuring a dog's cortisol level once is not very informa- tive. The levels fluctuate greatly on a minute to minute basis, and even if the thermostat is set on the whole higher on average, individual levels can vary widely. Diagnosis is therefore based on taking a baseline measurement and then either stimulating or suppressing the system to see how high or low the levels go.

The ACTH stimulation test is accomplished by taking a blood sample for baseline cortisol level, injecting ACTH, and taking a second blood sample for cortisol assay in two hours. This ACTH stimulates the adrenal glands to release cortisol at the highest rate possible. If the amount released is sig- nificantly higher than normal, the diagnosis can be made. The diagnostic accuracy of this test is about 85% and this is the test usually used to monitor treatment. Some drawbacks are that dogs with iatrogenic Cushing's disease often don't stimulate because the problem is caused by administering too much cortisone, not the dog making too much. Also, up to half of the dogs with adrenal tumors fail to stimulate into the diagnostic range.

The low-dose dexamethasone suppression test is accomplished by taking a blood sample for a baseline cortisol value, injecting dexamethasone, and measuring cortisol levels at intervals over an 8-hour period. The most important time interval is 6–8 hours, but a sample taken at 3–4 hours is some- times also helpful. The test is based on the premise that giving corticosteroids to a normal animal pushes down the blood levels of cortisol by negative feed- back just as a fire in the fireplace will turn off the furnace by its effecton the thermostat. Since animals with Cushing's disease have a higher "thermo- stat" setting, the cortisols in these animals are less suppressed by the admin- istration of corticosteroids. The test is considered about 90% diagnostic, and normal dogs show significant suppression of cortisol levels for at least 8 hours, whereas dogs with Cushing's disease have levels that have recovered by that time, even if they suppressed initially.

Combinations of the dexamethasone suppression test and the ACTH stimulation test are sometimes advocated in hard-to-diagnose cases and were originally thought to help predict the location of the problem to within the brain or the adrenals. There is some debate among endocrinologists as to whether the combination test can actually provide this information and, in general, other tests are superior at demonstrating the actual location of the problem.

The reason it is necessary to determine whether a dog has pituitary disease (85%) or adrenal disease (15%) is not just academic interest — pituitary disease is treated with medicines and adrenal disease is treated with surgery. The principal test used to distinguish betweenthe two is the high-dose dexametha-sone suppression test. The test works similar to the low-dose dexamethasone suppression test but a much higher dose of corticosteroid is given. The premise is that tumors in the adrenals are more resistant to suppression by cortico-steroid than are tumors in the pituitary. Of course, this test should only be used in animals in which the diagnosis of Cushing's disease has already been made. This test should be used cautiously in diabetic animals since ketoacido-sis, a serious complication of diabetes, can result from the higher dosage of corticosteroid administered in this test.

Other tests have also been proposed to help make the distinction but are not available from all diagnostic laboratories. A test that measures the actual plasma concentration of ACTH is helpful because low levels would be suggestive of adrenal tumors and high levels of pituitary disease; this is being evaluated at many veterinary colleges and veterinary laboratories. The test is currently available from a small number of specialized facilities. The metyrapone suppression test is based on the premise that metyrapone sup-presses an enzyme important in converting an intermediate substance (11-DOC) to cortisol. Elevated levels of 11-DOC suggest pituitary disease and little or no change suggests adrenal tumor.

It is not always necessary to determine the ultimate cause of the disease. If owners are completely unwilling to consider surgery (and this sometimes happens), medical therapy can be instituted without additional laboratory work and, about 85% of the time, the condition will be controlled. Also, radiographs (x-rays), ultrasound examination, or computed tomography (CT) scans may identify an abdominal tumor in the area of the adrenal gland.

Treatment

Even though Cushing's disease is frequently caused by a tumor in either the brain or the abdomen, there are a number of successful treatment options available. In people, both causes are treated surgically, but there are very few facilities capable of performing pituitary microsurgery in dogs. The most common cause, a pituitary tumor, is treated in dogs with a medication called o',p'-DDD (mitotane or Lysodren), which selectively poisons the adrenal gland and causes it to release less cortisol. It is usually given daily, with food, for the first week, then once a week thereafter. Too much medication is poten-tially quite dangerous, so monitoring cortisol levels is important. If there are any side effects (vomiting, diarrhea, awkwardness) caused by pushing the cortisol levels too low, small amounts of cortisone can be given on those days or the treatment dose of o',p'-DDD altered. ACTH stimulation tests should be performed after 3 months initially (earlier if warranted), and then every 6–12 months to monitor the condition. As dogs are maintained for months and years, the dosage often needs to be increased and the interval may need to be shortened to twice weekly or even daily. This happens because some dogs become more resistant to mitotane with long-term use; changes are made if cortisol values continue to climb while on therapy.

Another potential treatment for pituitary-dependent Cushing's disease is ketoconazole, a drug more commonly used to treat deep fungal infections. It just so happens that one of the potential side effects of ketoconazole is lowering blood levels of cortisol, which is a positive effect in dogs with Cushing's disease. It can also be used to stabilize dogs with adrenal tumors before surgery or in place of surgery should this option be declined by owners. The disadvantage is that the effect on cortisol levels is transient and so this somewhat expensive drug must be given twice daily for maintenance rather than once weekly.

Two other approaches to the pituitary-related disease are brain surgery and cobalt radiation therapy. The microsurgical approach to the pituitary gland is far more difficult in dogs than in people, and to date, not nearly as successful. The use of cobalt irradiation is usually reserved for dogs in which the tumor is pressing on other structures in the brain and causing neurological problems.

Adrenal tumors account for less than 15% of cases of Cushing's disease, and about half of those are malignant and half benign. The best treatment for adrenal tumors is their surgical removal, but the surgery is complicated by the fact that animals can go into shock when the cancerous gland is removed and their blood levels of cortisone drop precipitously. This is prevented by keeping dogs on fluids containing cortisone compounds before, during, and following surgery and then switching to oral corticosteroids for about a month until the other adrenal gland (which has been shriveled up because of inactivity compared to the tumor) has had time to recover and produce sufficient amounts of cortisol itself. Unfortunately, about half of all dogs surviving surgery eventually succumb to complications, including kidney failure, pneumonia, and thromboembolism. This is probably because they are released too soon from the hospital, but this is often a financial decision rather than a medical one. There is little doubt that it is quite expensive to keep a dog in intensive care for weeks after surgery.

GROWTH HORMONE-RESPONSIVE DERMATOSIS

Growth hormone-responsive dermatosis is a controversial and relatively new endocrine disease presumed to be due to decreased growth hormone levels in the blood. If an animal is deficient in growth hormone from birth, it becomes a dwarf. If it acquires a deficiency later in life, a pattern of hair loss develops that resembles that of other endocrine diseases, especially Cushing's disease. The disorder is controversial, because the evidence that the primary problem is related to growth hormone is not very convincing. Growth hormone is not regulated by the same thermostat-like negative feedback systems that control thyroid and adrenal hormones, but rather by intermediate insulin-like growth factors called somatomedins.

Growth hormone-responsive dermatosis is so named because it responds to treatment with growth hormone. But it also responds to other alternatives as well. In fact, much current research is focused on the possibility that the disorder is the result of overproduction of male sex hormones by the adrenal glands.

Males are much more commonly affected than females, and most affected animals are quite young, often 1–3 years of age. The condition is seen in various breeds, but those predisposed include the Chow Chow, Pomeranian, Poodle, Airedale, Samoyed, American Water Spaniel, and Keeshond. Dogs with this form of dermatosis start to lose hair on their trunks, but the legs and head remain relatively spared. In time, the skin often becomes quite dark in the areas of hair loss.

The diagnosis of this condition is not straightforward, because the ultimate cause has not been proven. Biopsies are often helpful but can't necessarily tell the difference between this and other endocrine disorders. Blood tests are typically taken that measure growth hormone, somatomedin, or sex hormone levels. Unfortunately, these specialized tests are only available from a few laboratories. The most common test is the growth hormone stimulation test in which growth hormone levels are measured before and after the injection of xylazine or human growth hormone-releasing factor. Affected animals typically have very low levels of growth hormone. Much research is currently being done on sex hormone levels in these dogs, especially the sex hormones that are produced by the adrenal glands such as dehydroepiandrosterone sulfate (DHEAS) and androstenedione. If this research is fruitful it will likely change our entire approach to diagnosis and treatment.

Treatment

Therapy of growth hormone-responsive dermatosis requires deliberation. Since the condition does not affect the health of the animal, treatment is only for cosmetic reasons. The hair loss doesn't bother the dog and doesn't carry any health risks, so doing nothing is something worth considering. Since male hormones appear to be involved in many cases, neutering is an excellent recommendation, especially in Chow Chows and Samoyeds, which respond especially well to this form of therapy.

When it comes to medical therapy, growth hormone is in short supply and relatively expensive. It is usually administered by injection twice weekly for six weeks or every other day for three weeks, and hair growth is expected within about three months. Treatment with growth hormone is not without risk; diabetes mellitus may result because of the effect on insulin levels. Therefore, blood glucose levels should be monitored throughout treatment.

Other proposed therapies include ketoconazole and Lysodren. Ketoconazole has been shown to affect sex hormone levels, so this is its likely mode of action. Lysodren is a potent toxin for the adrenal gland and is used in the treatment of Cushing's disease. It likely is effective by modifying the interaction of hormones at hair follicle receptors to stimulate hair follicle growth. Lysodren has been particularly helpful in Pomeranians, in which an adrenal enzyme deficiency has been documented. As we learn more about this disorder, treatment recommendations will undoubtedly change.

SEX HORMONE DISORDERS

Despite the fact that many different skin conditions are blamed on disorders of sex hormones, actual problems involving the common male and female sex hormones are relatively rare. These problems can result when levels are too high or too low.

Hyperestrogenism

Hyperestrogenism results when levels of the female sex hormone estrogen get too high in the bloodstream. This can occur due to functional cysts on the ovaries, ovarian cancers, or administration of estrogen-containing drugs to treat other conditions. This syndrome was previously referred to as ovarian imbalance type I. As there is in many other endocrine disorders, there is hair loss in this condition. It is usually around the genitals and extending down the hind legs. Often the vulva and nipples are swollen due to the high circulating levels of female sex hormones. Itchiness, waxy ears, and a greasy, scaly haircoat are frequently also part of this disorder, and heat cycles are irregular, prolonged, or suppressed. There may also be a history of previous endometritis or pyometra.

Diagnosis is made tentatively, since it is extremely difficult to identify any cysts or tumors without surgery or to measure abnormalities in blood levels of the common female sex hormones. Blood samples are usually collected to measure blood counts and estradiol levels. The blood counts are used to evaluate bone marrow function, and estradiol levels may be diagnostic in some, but not all, cases. The treatment of choice is ovariohysterectomy (spay), which is the complete removal of the uterus and ovaries. In a limited number of cases, drugs have been used that can destroy the cysts, but these products have not been licensed for this purpose. Also, the problem frequently recurs with the next heat. There may be a hereditary component to developing cystic ovaries. Treatment is important, because chronic elevation of estrogens in the blood may make the animal more susceptible to bone marrow suppression, inflammation in the uterus, and possibly mammary cancers.

Estrogen-Responsive Dermatosis

Estrogen-responsive dermatosis, formerly known as ovarian imbalance type II, is presumed to occur when blood levels of estrogen are too low. It has never been documented, however, that dogs with this condition are really deficient in estrogen. It is usually seen in older females that were spayed at an early age. Dachshunds and Boxers seem to be affected most often. The condition is very similar to hyperestrogenism, except that the nipples and vulva are infantile in appearance. Dribbling of urine (urinary incontinence) is common. Diagnosis is based on the history, clinical examination, and response to estrogen supplementation. Estrogens should be used cautiously because of possible suppression of the bone marrow.

Tumors of the Testicles

Tumors of the testicles can sometimes secrete female sex hormones and result in hyperestrogenism in male dogs. The incidence of this condition is much higher in dogs whose testicles have not descended completely from the abdominal cavity into the scrotum (cryptorchidism). The syndrome is characterized by hair loss around the rear end, without inflammation, enlargement of the mammary glands (gynecomastia), drooping of the prepuce, and other signs of feminization. Affected male dogs may squat to urinate, attract other male dogs, have a decreased sex drive, and even produce milk from the enlarged mammary glands. Diseases of the prostate gland and estrogen-induced bone marrow suppression are possible consequences of the disorder. Diagnosis is based on the history, physical examination, and response to castration. Since about 10% of these tumors are malignant and may metastasize (spread), chest x-rays and blood tests should be considered before castration.

Castration-Responsive Dermatosis

Castration-responsive dermatosis is a strange disorder that involves hair loss on the neck and trunk without feminization or testicular tumors. The skin is often dry and gets progressively darker. It has been reported in the Chow Chow and Shetland Sheepdog. These dogs have no actual diagnosable disease, but their hair regrows following castration.

Woolly Syndrome

Woolly syndrome has been reported in Siberian Huskies, Malamutes, and Keeshonden. Dogs with this condition develop typical endocrine patterns of hair loss on the back, perineum, and the backs of the hind legs. The remaining hair on the trunk is dry, brittle, or crimped (woolly). In some cases, the coat even changes to a bronze color. These animals also respond to castration by regrowing normal hair in two to three months.

Hypertestosteronemia

Hypertestosteronemia is associated with high blood levels of testosterone caused most often by a functional tumor on the testicles. The skin around the anus and genitals becomes dark, greasy, and thickened, and the tail gland (an oval region on the top of the tail) may get larger and lose its hair covering. The condition responds to neutering, by removing the cancerous testicle.

Testosterone-Responsive Dermatosis

Testosterone-responsive dermatosis is an exceptionally rare disease, suspected to occur in old male dogs. There is a patterned hair loss and the remaining hair is dry or dull. Because the symptoms can be very similar to male hyperestrogenism and both may have symptoms due to a hormonal imbalance, accurate diagnosis is often difficult. In general, if dogs have the symptoms and they are intact, castration is worthwhile. If they have already been castrated, options include supplementation with testosterone or doing nothing. Since testosterone administration can have several side effects, including liver disease, keratinization disorders, and aggressive behavior, conscientious neglect is worth considering.

Hormonal Hypersensitivity

Hormonal hypersensitivity is quite a rare hormonal problem in which dogs develop allergic reactions to the hormones they produce. It is most commonly seen in females, especially those with a history of pseudopregnancy or irregular "heat" cycles. Males are only occasionally affected. In females, the condition starts as an itchy rash around the hind end that usually occurs during estrus (heat) or pseudopregnancy. In time the itchiness becomes prolonged and continuous; often the nipples and vulva become enlarged from repeated trauma. When males are affected, the itchiness is constant from the outset. The diagnosis may be confirmed by performing a modified allergy test in which estrogen, progesterone, and testosterone are injected into the dermis and the response evaluated in fifteen minutes and again in forty-eight hours. The itchiness is usually dramatically reduced within ten days of neutering.

8

SKIN TUMORS

Skin tumors are the most common form of cancer seen in dogs. There are many different kinds of skin cancer in dogs, and in people, and to sort them out, it is important to understand the "lingo" applied to cancer. Only when we all speak the same language can cancer be truly understood.

The science of cancer is referred to as oncology, and medical specialists dealing with cancer patients are called oncologists. Many terms are used in place of cancer, including neoplasia, tumor, and growth, but none of these, on its own, is really any more descriptive. We may say an animal has a neoplasm (new growth), but that doesn't tell us if it is harmful. Similarly, an animal with a tumor or growth may have a serious disease or a harmless nubbin.

Most cancers originate from specific cells of the body. We use the term "skin cancer" loosely, but there are no "skin cells" as such, and therefore skin cancer is a very general term for any growth that involves any of the cell types found in the skin. Thus, cancers might derive from any of the different cells of the epidermis, hair follicles, glands, fibrous tissue, blood vessels, mast cells, white blood cells, pigment-producing cells, or even the fat. All of these could be called skin cancers, and yet all are distinct. The one thing that all cancers have in common is that their rate of growth is uncontrolled. This alone, however, is not cause for alarm.

Not all skin tumors are harmful; most owners are familiar with the harmless lumps and bumps seen on many dogs. To tell the difference, a method of naming tumors has evolved that describes the nature of the cancer and its risk to the animal. Benign tumors are unlikely to have complications and are designated by the suffix -oma (e.g., lipoma, a benign fatty tumor). Malignant tumors do much harm and may also metastasize (spread). If their origin is surface epithelium, they are designated by the suffix -carcinoma (e.g., adenocarcinoma, a malignant glandular cancer). If they are nonepithelial, they are given the suffix -sarcoma (e.g., liposarcoma, a malignant fatty tumor). Surface epithelium lines not only the skin but the digestive tract, glands, reproductive tract, and respiratory system. The nonepithelial tissues include bones, cartilage, fibrous tissue, fat, and blood cells.

Most tumors are diagnosed by removing them in part or completely and submitting samples to pathologists. If an appropriate sample is collected, a diagnosis can often be made and comments provided to suggest if the growth was completely removed or not. Whenever possible, the pathologist also tries to provide a prognosis, a best guess for the likely outcome of the problem. This prognosis is based on the outcome of previous cases with the same condition. The prognosis given by the pathologist is not meant to be taken as absolute fact; it is only a guideline. The prognosis with skin tumors varies from good to poor, depending on the type of neoplasm involved.

Another quick test that is frequently done with tumors is called cytology. This is often accomplished by taking an "aspirate," which involves sucking tumor cells into a needle syringe and expressing the contents onto a microscope slide. If tumors are completely or partially removed, an edge can be touched to a microscope slide as well, and this is referred to as an "impression smear." Cytology works better for some tumors than for others, but it may offer a quick diagnosis; biopsy results may take days or weeks. But even if a preliminary diagnosis can be made by cytology, it is always best to also do a biopsy, because these provide important clues to the "architecture" of the tumor and allow for a more informed prognosis.

When it comes to treatment of skin cancers, there are many options. If there is a single tumor, it is best to remove it entirely so that diagnosis and treatment can be accomplished at the same time. This surgical procedure is excision, "cutting out" the tumor. Other forms of surgery may use supercold liquids (cryosurgery), electric currents (electrosurgery), or heat (hyperthermia) to destroy the tumor cells. Medicines used to treat cancers are usually grouped under the heading chemotherapy, the use of chemicals or drugs to treat disease. Most of these medicines work by poisoning rapidly growing cells. Since cancer cells grow faster than normal cells, they are more affected by these substances. Radiation therapy is also used in the treatment of skin cancers, although some cancers are more successfully treated than others. Finally, immunotherapy remains a goal for the future—using the immune system to target and get rid of cancer cells. This has been used on a limited basis for the treatment of mast-cell tumors and some breast cancers. Unfortunately, some products, such as interferon, have not turned out to be the cancer cures the press had predicted, but they do represent important advances.

Over the years it has been found that certain breeds of dogs are more prone to certain cancers than others. Some cancers are more common in males, while others are more common in females. This doesn't mean that the cancers are inherited; rather, there is a breed tendency, or more commonly a breed predisposition. Don't be alarmed! The statistics only mean that certain breeds have a higher relative risk of developing certain cancers—it certainly does not imply that these breeds will necessarily get these cancers or that they are not prone to developing others.

BASAL-CELL TUMOR

Basal-cell tumors are common benign growths that may be most commonly seen in Poodles and Cocker Spaniels. The tumors are found predominantly in middle-aged dogs (average is 9 years of age). Basal-cell tumors may develop on sun-damaged skin, though this has not been decidedly proven. They are more commonly found on the head, neck, and shoulders. Diagnosis is made by biopsy. The tumors may be surgically removed or left without problem.

BASOSQUAMOUS CARCINOMA

This is a rare tumor, perhaps a malignant relative of the basal-cell tumor. It is quite aggressive and can spread to the lymph nodes and lungs. Early surgical intervention is important, since this tumor has been known to recur if not completely removed.

CYSTS

Cutaneous cysts are very common. They are actually parts of the skin, hair follicles, or glands that form enclosed capsules in the dermis or subcutaneous fat. There are many different types, including apocrine cysts, dermoid cysts, epidermal cysts, follicular cysts, and proliferating follicular cysts. All of these cysts are benign and can be effectively cured with surgery. The diagnosis is made by biopsy.

FIBROMA

Fibromas are uncommon benign tumors, seen more frequently in females and with a breed predisposition for Boxers, Boston Terriers, and Fox Terriers.

Older animals are affected most often, and the lumps are mostly seen on the skin of the legs, flanks, and genital area. They occur singly rather than in crops and may be firm or soft. They can be completely removed by surgery, and diagnosis is confirmed by biopsy.

FIBROSARCOMA

Fibrosarcomas are the malignant counterpart of fibromas. They, too, are more common in females and may have a predilection for Cocker Spaniels. The average age of affected dogs is about 9 years. These malignancies are often irregular in shape and may ulcerate on the surface of the skin. They are most commonly found on the legs and trunk, less often on the head, neck, mouth, and mammary regions. Fibrosarcomas are easily diagnosed, but treatment is often quite difficult. If the tumors are not completely removed surgically, they recur in about 30% of cases. Radiation, hyperthermia, and even arterial cross-circulation (a special type of transfusion) have been proposed as alternative forms of therapy for fibrosarcoma. A new product, called acemannan, has recently been released. It is a natural immune stimulant derived from the aloe plant.

GENERALIZED NODULAR DERMATOFIBROSIS

Generalized nodular dermatofibrosis has been observed in German Shepherd Dogs in association with kidney cancers and is more completely described in the chapter on breed-related disorders. The skin lumps are not dangerous themselves but are an indicator of an increased risk for specific cancers inside, especially a tumor of the kidneys known as renal cystadenocarcinoma. Treatment of the skin tumors is usually not necessary unless they begin to interfere with movement. Most attention is focused on checking for internal cancers of the kidney and/or uterus.

GRANULOMATOUS SKIN DISEASES

Granulomatous skin diseases are not tumors but are included here because they are often suspected to be tumors until biopsies are evaluated.

Granulomas are inflammatory conditions in which the body tries to "wall off" substances, using specialized white blood cells known as histiocytes.

Microbial granulomas are not uncommon and have been reported for staphylococci, mycobacteria, dermatophytosis, intermediate and systemic fungi, pythiosis, algae, and a variety of other microorganisms. All are diagnosed by biopsy, and special staining procedures are often required to highlight and identify the microbes. Treatment is difficult because most antibiotics do not penetrate granulomas well.

Parasitic granulomas can occur with a variety of parasites, including heartworm and *Leishmania*. Tick bites can also result in granulomas. Treatment must be directed specifically at the parasite. Corticosteroids are often necessary to reduce the inflammation in tick-bite granulomas.

Eosinophilic granuloma is seen most commonly in Siberian Huskies and is covered in more detail in the chapter on immune-mediated skin diseases. It usually responds well to intermediate doses of corticosteroids.

Sterile pyogranuloma is also covered in the chapter on immune-mediated skin diseases. It often causes lumps between the toes or on the face of a dog. The cause is unknown, but because the growths respond to drugs that suppress the immune system, there is probably an immunologic connection.

Granulomatous sebaceous adenitis is a granulomatous disease that targets the hair follicles and the sebaceous glands that supply them. Because some, but not all, cases respond to such different therapies as corticosteroids, retinoids, and cyclosporine, it is suspected that probably several different diseases are currently being labeled sebaceous adenitis. The condition is described more fully in the chapter on keratinization disorders.

Sterile nodular panniculitis, also known as juvenile panniculitis, is an uncommon condition described in the chapter on immune-mediated skin diseases. It occurs in young dogs, especially Dachshunds and Miniature Poodles, and responds completely to as little as two weeks' worth of corticosteroids. The cause is unknown, but a transient immunologic disease is suspected.

Histiocytic syndromes are discussed below and include cutaneous histiocytosis, malignant histiocytosis, and fibrous histiocytoma. They are suspected of being inflammatory diseases rather than cancers, but their causes are still the matter of much speculation.

Sterile sarcoidal granulomatous skin disease is very rare indeed, but cases have been reported in the Great Dane, Shetland Sheepdog, and Irish Setter. Lumps appear predominantly on the neck and trunk but are usually neither painful nor itchy. Diagnosis is made by biopsy, and the condition often responds well to corticosteroids.

Xanthomas are caused by abnormalities in lipid (fat) metabolism and cause small bumps in which inflammatory cells in the skin are loaded with lipid droplets. It can occur as a congenital disease or be the result of other diseases, such as diabetes mellitus.

HEMANGIOMA

Hemangiomas (cherry tumors) are uncommon benign tumors of blood vessels. The average age of affected dogs is about 8 years. Boxers may be at increased risk. The tumors usually arise singly and occur most commonly on the legs, flanks, neck, and face. Although the tumors cause no real concern, they are sometimes removed, because their rich blood supply may result in bleeding if the area is injured.

HEMANGIOSARCOMA

Hemangiosarcoma is the malignant variant of hemangioma and occurs most commonly in males. On average, these growths are seen in dogs that are about 8 years old. German Shepherd Dogs, Boxers, and Bernese Mountain Dogs seem most often affected. Although hemangiosarcomas can arise from blood vessels of the skin, they are most commonly associated with cancers of the spleen and the right atrium of the heart. If these internal tumors rupture, there can be profound blood loss, collapse, shock, and even death. The growths are highly invasive and malignant and spread easily because of their rich blood supply. Treatment is difficult, and the prognosis is often poor to guarded. In dogs with primary cancer of the spleen, removal of the spleen (splenectomy) is an important aspect of treatment.

HEMANGIOPERICYTOMA

Hemangiopericytomas are common benign tumors thought to originate from the tissue surrounding blood vessels. Boxers, German Shepherd Dogs, Cocker Spaniels, Springer Spaniels, and Fox Terriers appear predisposed. Females are more commonly affected than males. These tumors can get very large; they occur most commonly on the legs, but are occasionally found on the trunk, head, neck, and mammary regions. The average age of affected dogs is about 9 years. Surgery is an effective treatment, but about a quarter of the tumors eventually return. Radiation therapy may be useful when complete excision is not possible.

HISTIOCYTOMA

Histiocytomas (button tumors) are fairly common tumors, most often seen in dogs less than 2 years old. Histiocytomas are more prevalent in the

Boxer, Cocker Spaniel, Great Dane, Shetland Sheepdog, and Dachshund but may occur in any breed. The tumors may be induced by a virus, but this remains unsubstantiated. They are small, red, often singular, and usually occur on the head, ears, or legs. Diagnosis can be easily made by biopsy, but care must be used in the selection of pathologists. Since this tumor does not occur in people, pathologists unfamiliar with veterinary medicine may call it a malignant cutaneous histiocytoma and recomend aggressive treatment. In dogs, this tumor will eventually regress spontaneously if not removed surgically. Only rarely do new tumors arise at the site of excision or at other sites.

HISTIOCYTOMA, FIBROUS

Nodular fasciitis was originally referred to as fibrous histiocytoma, but it now appears that this is an inflammatory disease rather than a cancer. This disorder affects young (2–4 years of age on average) Collies preferentially, causing reddish lumps on the eyelids and lips. Most ophthalmologists refer to the condition as nodular (granulomatous) episcleritis. Diagnosis is made by biopsy, and most cases respond to injections of corticosteroids. In unresponsive cases, azathioprine is an alternative.

HISTIOCYTOMA, MALIGNANT FIBROUS

Malignant fibrous histiocytoma is rare. It is locally invasive but slow to spread. One of its manifestations is also known as giant cell tumor, a condition in which more than one cell has fused together to form a giant cell with more than one nucleus. It is seen most often on the legs and neck but is so rare that generalizations are difficult to make. The diagnosis is made by biopsy, and the most appropriate treatment is complete surgical excision.

HISTIOCYTOSIS, CUTANEOUS

Cutaneous histiocytosis differs from histiocytoma in that numerous lumps occur, wax and wane, and appear in new sites, regardless of treatment. Like fibrous histiocytoma, this appears to be more an inflammatory disease than a cancer, and internal spread does not occur. Diagnosis is made by biopsy, and treatment is often attempted with corticosteroids and chemotherapy, although they are only temporarily beneficial.

HISTIOCYTOSIS, MALIGNANT

Malignant histiocytosis occurs most commonly in the Bernese Mountain Dog, in which it follows a rapidly progressive and inevitably fatal course. Multiple lumps are distributed on the body surface, but occur most commonly on the scrotum, nose, and eyelids. Affected dogs lose energy, have weight loss and trouble breathing, as well as enlarged lymph nodes, liver, and spleen. In most cases the cancer principally involves the lungs. The diagnosis is made by biopsy, and all forms of therapy have been ineffective. Since the cell involved, the histiocyte, is an important cell of the immune system, immuno-modulation remains an option worth attempting. Much more research is needed before any true recommendations can be made.

INTRACUTANEOUS CORNIFYING EPITHELIOMA

Intracutaneous cornifying epithelioma (also known as keratoacanthoma) usually develops in younger dogs (less than 5 years of age), and males are more often affected than females. In most breeds the tumors occur singly with a pore on the surface, but in such breeds as the Norwegian Elkhound, Old English Sheepdog, and Keeshond they may be multiple, ranging in number from a few growths to several hundred. For single tumors, surgery usually cures the condition. Care should be taken not to squeeze these tumors, because they may rupture, causing much irritation to the skin. Since they are not harmful, even multiple tumors may be left without treatment. Some of the newer vitamin A derivatives such as etretinate (Tegison) have successfully been used to treat generalized keratoacanthomas in people and have also been somewhat beneficial in dogs, although the product is currently not licensed for this use.

KERATOSES

Keratoses are accumulations of keratin, the surface scale of skin. Depending on their content, they may be referred to as seborrheic, actinic, lichenoid, or proliferative keratoses. These are discussed in the chapter on keratinization disorders.

LIPOMA

Lipomas are common benign tumors arising from subcutaneous fat. They are most common in older dogs (8 years average). Obese dogs may be predisposed to these tumors, and females are affected more often thanmales; Cocker Spaniels, Dachshunds, Weimaraners, Labrador Retrievers, and terriers appear to be most at risk. These lumps are usually soft and flabby and are most often found around the neck, chest, abdomen, and legs. Most lipomas cause no problems, although they can get quite large. In general, lipomas can be neglected, but some that compromise the function of other organ systems or are a nuisance to the animal may be surgically removed. Putting the dog on a diet beforehand not only lessens the risk of surgery, but also helps delineate the tumor. An alternative to surgery has been suggested in which calcium chloride is injected into the tumor to destroy the fat cells. With this treatment, the skin overlying the lipoma may also become compromised and slough.

LIPOSARCOMA

Liposarcomas are rare malignant variants of the common lipoma. It is important to understand that these cancers do not arise from existing lipomas. They are independent tumors that grow rapidly and invade but are slow to spread by metastasis. Surgery is the best treatment, but chemotherapy may be necessary if the entire tumor cannot be excised.

LIPOMATOSIS, INFILTRATIVE

Infiltrative lipomas, or lipomatosis, is a proliferative disease of fat cells that go on to infiltrate or replace muscle or collagen. They can interfere with movement and are difficult to remove entirely but are very slow to metastasize.

LYMPHOSARCOMA

Cutaneous lymphosarcoma is a malignant disorder of lymphocytes. Since lymphocytes develop into many different cells, there are many different forms of lymphosarcoma that can arise from those cells.

Cutaneous lymphosarcoma can occur strictly as a skin disease, or it can be a cancer involving many different internal organs. B-cell lymphosarcoma is more common in elderly dogs, with males three times more frequently affected than females. In addition to skin disease, affected dogs may also have leukemia, or involvement of the liver, spleen, lungs, and lymph nodes. Strictly cutaneous B-cell lymphosarcoma is quite rare. In addition to biopsies, diagnosis should include a variety of blood tests and radiographs (x-rays) to search for internal involvement. Treatment of B-cell lymphosarcoma is usually attempted with corticosteroids and combination chemotherapy using several anticancer drugs (e.g., cyclophosphamide, azathioprine, vincristine, L-asparaginase, doxorubicin, chlorambucil).

Cutaneous T-cell-like lymphoma (mycosis fungoides) is a slightly less malignant condition that evolves from a red scaly rash (erythroderma) through a plaque stage to large cutaneous lumps. This evolution may occur over months or years; Cocker Spaniels and Poodles appear to be affected most often. The condition is most important, because in its early stages, it doesn't look like a cancer at all and may be improperly diagnosed as eczema, seborrhea, or allergy. Diagnosis is made by biopsy, but very early cases may be hard to confirm.

Treatment of T-cell lymphomas can be undertaken with the realization that, for the most part, by the time a diagnosis is made, the tumor has already spread. So far, it does not appear that treatment increases survival time, although animals certainly look better with treatment. Since T-cell lymphoma evolves slowly over months and years, animals usually survive for a considerable period whether treated or not. When treatment is needed, corticosteroids and topical mechlorethamine (nitrogen mustard) may be of some benefit. Combination chemotherapy may be beneficial for T-cell lymphomas, as it is for B-cell lymphomas. An additional form of therapy has been reported that involves daily intradermal injections of a solution of placental lysate, but this has yet to be extensively studied.

Pagetoid reticulosis, or Woringer-Kolopp disease, is a rare disorder with some features similar to T-cell lymphoma. It has been reported to involve the mouth and footpads, but too few cases have been reported to draw any real conclusions. It is diagnosed and treated similarly to T-cell lymphoma.

MAMMARY TUMORS

Mammary tumors (tumors of the breast) are common in dogs, but most are preventable. Bitches spayed before their first heat are more than 99% less likely to develop mammary cancer than intact bitches. The risk becomes equal when bitches are allowed to have more than four heats before they are neutered. Therefore, neutering at the time of tumor evaluation or removal will not affect the survival time of affected bitches.

Dogs have a higher incidence of mammary cancer than do other domestic animals or women (three times the incidence of breast cancer in women). About 60% of all mammary tumors in dogs are in the fourth or fifth mammary glands, which are thought to be the most hormonally active. Not all breast lumps are cancerous, of course, but of those that are tumors, about half are benign and half malignant. Those that are malignant are quick to spread to other glands and lymph nodes and to the lungs, skin, liver, kidney, heart, bone, and brain. Diagnosis is best made by biopsy, since cytology (the evaluation of individual cells) is quicker but not as accurate.

Some benign mammary tumors are thought to become malignant with time, so all mammary lumps should be surgically removed. At the time of excision, the surgeon should carefully examine the lymph nodes for signs of involvement. The entire mammary gland and surrounding tissue is removed if localized spread is anticipated. Prior to surgery, chest x-rays, blood counts, and biochemical profiles are performed. If spread is evident internally, surgery is unlikely to be very helpful. Radiation therapy may be helpful in preventing local recurrence of tumors if they haven't metastasized. Very little information is available on use of chemotherapy and immunotherapy in canine mammary tumors, and even less on antiestrogen hormonal treatments. These are therapies that may prove helpful to dogs as well as women in the future.

MAST-CELL TUMORS

Mast-cell tumors are relatively common in dogs that are about 8 years old. They are most prevalent in Boxers, Boston Terriers, English Bulldogs, Bull Terriers, Fox Terriers, Staffordshire Terriers, Labrador Retrievers, Dachshunds, and Weimaraners. Both sexes are equally affected. The tumors are more common on the trunk, anogenital region, and legs but can appear elsewhere. Although these tumors may either act benign or malignant, all mast-cell tumors should be treated as being potentially malignant; those affecting the anogenital area and toes usually are. Since mast cells contain many active substances, including histamine and heparin, other problems may be noted in dogs with mast-cell tumors. Some may have intestinal bleeding or a lack of blood clotting. With systemic mastocytosis, the spread of malignant mast cells internally can cause anorexia, vomiting, and diarrhea in about half of affected dogs. The lymph nodes, spleen, and liver are most commonly involved.

Mast-cell tumors are usually easy to diagnose because the cancerous mast cells are abundant and easy to recover and identify. Mast-cell tumors can be easily diagnosed by cytology, but this does not allow them to be graded; biopsies should still be submitted for histopathologic examination. Biopsy specimens of mast-cell tumors are often graded by the pathologist to help form a prognosis. Very recently it has been proposed that the clinical grading for mast-cell tumors be changed to reflect that used by pathologists. Grade I tumors are well-differentiated and the most common form of tumor in dogs. Only about 10% of dogs with Grade I mast-cell tumors die as a result of metastasis or inoperable recurrence. Grade II tumors are usually larger, deeper, and less well-circumscribed. They account for about 25% of mast-cell tumors in dogs and 45% of dogs will die as a direct result of these tumors. Grade III mast-cell tumors are rare and are usually large, ulcerated and poorly circumscribed. About 85% of dogs die from these tumors.

Single tumors are best treated by surgery, while multiple tumors usually require some form of chemotherapy. Cryosurgery (freezing tissues with super-cold liquids) has been useful, especially for multiple small skin tumors. A wide margin of normal tissue around the tumor must be frozen to lessen the chance of recurrence. Radiation therapy is an effective treatment of mast-cell tumor in dogs and is usually administered three times per week for a total of ten equal treatments. As a final alternative, injections directly into the tumor of preparations of *Proprionibacterium acnes* (ImmunoRegulin) or mycobacteria (Regressin) may stimulate the dog's immune response and result in the tumor shrinking somewhat after 3–4 months. Corticosteroids are also frequently used in dogs with mast-cell tumors to counteract the sub-stances released by the tumor cells, and cimetidine, an ulcer medication, is given when animals are experiencing gastrointestinal bleeding.

MELANOMA

Melanomas are tumors of the pigment-producing melanocytes. They may be benign or malignant. Scottish Terriers, Boston Terriers, Airedale Terriers, Cocker Spaniels, Boxers, Irish Setters, Chow Chows, Chihuahuas, and Springer Spaniels have a higher incidence of melanomas than other breeds. Males appear to be affected more often than females. The tumors arise most commonly around the mouth, genitals, and mammary glands. As a general rule, those arising on skin are more likely to be benign than those originating on mucous membranes.

Melanomas are diagnosed by pathologists, but there is not always a clear-cut distinction between benign and malignant tumors. It is uncommon for benign melanomas to convert to malignant forms, but since it is impossible to guarantee that a melanoma is benign, all melanomas should be entirely removed surgically.

MYXOMA

Myxomas are rare tumors related to fibromas. They are more common in older dogs and occur most commonly on the legs, back, and groin. This tumor tends to infiltrate surrounding tissues, so it may recur following surgery if all of the tumor was not removed.

MYXOSARCOMA

Myxosarcomas are the malignant counterparts of the myxoma and can spread (albeit rarely) to the lungs and other tissues. They are diagnosed by biopsy, but it is not always an easy matter to differentiate from malignant varieties. They are treated similarly to fibrosarcomas.

NEVI

A nevus (cutaneous hamartoma) is a localized developmental skin defect. The cells that form the nevus determine its classification (sebaceous nevus, collagen nevus, epidermal nevus, etc.). Some are more important than others. Collagenous nevi are particularly important because they may be difficult to differentiate from nodular dermatofibrosis. They are most commonly seen in German Shepherd Dogs. Melanocytic nevi are important because they may be confused with melanoma. Therefore, nevi are harmless disorders that can mimic certain cancers. Most nevi are diagnosed when surgically removed tissue, thought to be a tumor, is submitted to pathologists for accurate diagnosis.

PAPILLOMA

Cutaneous papillomas (warts) are skin tumors that usually occur as small, single, cauliflower-like nodules on the head, feet, and genitals of middle-aged to older dogs. They are not caused by viruses. Most tumors called papillomas or warts are usually neither. Misdiagnosed papillomas are most likely to be localized collections of sebaceous glands, referred to as sebaceous gland hyperplasia. Diagnosis of papillomas is made by biopsy, and these tumors can be removed or left in place.

PAPILLOMATOSIS

Viral papillomatosis is a different disorder than cutaneous papilloma. It is caused by a virus and results in proliferative growths in the mouths of young dogs. Biopsies needed for diagnosis will also often show evidence of viral involvement. Treatment is usually unnecessary, as most cases spontaneously regress. If needed, a "wart vaccine" can be formulated to hasten the process, but since the condition generally clears up on its own, this canine papillomatosis vaccine is not usually recommended. Some evidence suggests that the vaccine can induce cancers at the site of injection.

PERIANAL (HEPATOID-GLAND) ADENOMA

The hepatoid glands are modified sebaceous glands that are found around the anus, genitals, tailhead, and hind legs. The benign tumor that arises in these areas is therefore referred to as a perianal adenoma or hepatoid-gland adenoma. Hepatoid-gland adenomas are quite common and occur with greater frequency in males than in females. Cocker Spaniels, English Bulldogs, Samoyeds, and Beagles appear to get them most often. They are seen most frequently in animals over 8 years old and are easily diagnosed with a biopsy. Since the growth of these tumors is influenced by the male sex hormone testosterone, castrating the dog or injecting the tumor with the female sex hormone diethylstilbestrol (DES) usually shrinks the tumor enough so that it can be entirely removed by surgery. The tumor may recur in about a third of cases, especially if castration was not performed. Surgery must be carefully performed to avoid damage to sensitive nerves in this region, including the anal sphincter.

PERIANAL (HEPATOID-GLAND) ADENOCARCINOMA

Hepatoid-gland adenocarcinomas are the malignant counterparts of the perianal adenoma. They tend to grow more rapidly, ulcerate, and spread widely. They are diagnosed by biopsy and require aggressive treatment. Unfortunately, internal spread is common. Surgery should be attempted if there is no evidence of spread, and radiation therapy may also be warranted.

PILOMATRIXOMA

Pilomatrixomas are benign tumors originating from specialized hair-forming cells. They usually occur singly and may be found on the shoulders, back, flanks, or legs. Kerry Blue Terriers and Poodles appear to develop them more often than other breeds. Diagnosis is made by biopsy and surgery almost always takes care of the problem. Rarely, malignant varieties do occur.

PLASMACYTOMA

Plasma cells are lymphocytes that have evolved to produce antibodies. Although most plasmacytomas are considered benign, some are not. Cutaneous plasmacytomas occur as dome-shaped nodules seen mostly on the lips, trunk, toes, and ears. They are relatively benign. Mucocutaneous plasmacytomas occur on the mucous membranes of the mouth and rectum and can be malignant. This distinction may not be easily made by biopsy. Cutaneous plasmacytomas should be surgically removed, but mucocutaneous plasmacytomas may also require treatments similar to those used for lymphosarcoma.

SEBACEOUS-GLAND ADENOMA

Benign sebaceous-gland tumors are common in dogs and are seen mostly in animals over 9 years old. They are most frequently reported in Cocker Spaniels, Poodles, Beagles, Dachshunds, and Boston Terriers, and slightly more often in females. Benign sebaceous adenomas and benign sebaceous adenomatous hyperplasia are far more common than the malignant adenocarcinomas. Most benign sebaceous growths are misdiagnosed as warts but have the same good prognosis. They normally appear as small, lobed, sometimes greasy nodules and are most prevalent on the abdomen, chest, legs, head, neck, shoulders, eyelids, and ears. These tumors can be removed or left without treatment.

SEBACEOUS-GLAND CARCINOMA

Sebaceous-gland carcinomas are much rarer than their benign counterparts. The average age of dogs that develop them is 9 years, and Cocker Spaniels may be affected most often. Most tumors are located on the head, chest, abdomen, and front legs. These tumors grow rapidly and frequently ulcerate, but they do not usually metastasize. They are diagnosed by biopsy and can usually be completely removed by surgery. Local recurrence is possible if the tumor was not completely removed.

SQUAMOUS-CELL CARCINOMA

Squamous-cell carcinomas are the most malignant epithelial tumors of canine skin. Some of these occur as a result of chronic sun exposure. The Scottish Terrier, Pekingese, Boxer, Poodle, and Norwegian Elkhound may develop them more often than other breeds. The tumors are most commonly located on the limbs, trunk, head, and neck. Involvement of the toes is thought to be the most malignant form. Most squamous-cell carcinomas are locally invasive, but some, like those affecting the toes, are quick to metastasize to the lymph nodes and lungs. When the affected area is completely removed, the prognosis is usually good. For squamous-cell carcinomas of the toes and those showing aggressive features in biopsy results, the prognosis becomes more guarded. Therapy with platinum compounds (e.g., cisplatin), hyperthermia, cryosurgery, electrosurgery, and radiation therapy may also be used with more or less success.

SWEAT-GLAND TUMORS

The sebaceous glands may often be involved in tumors, but the apocrine and eccrine sweat glands only rarely become cancerous. Apocrine adenomas are most common in male dogs over the age of 8, and perhaps most frequently in Cocker Spaniels. The tumors are most frequently reported on the head and neck, and they can usually be cured by surgery.

Apocrine-gland adenocarcinomas are quite rare; they are most commonly found on the back, flanks, and feet. Removing them surgically is the best treatment, but they may return. Site irradiation should be contemplated if there is doubt as to whether the tumor was completely removed. Apocrine adenocarcinomas can metastasize to local lymph nodes and the lungs.

Eccrine adenomas are very rare and limited to the footpads, the only part of the dog's body in which these glands are prevalent. The malignant variant, clear-cell hidradenocarcinoma, is exceptionally rare. Too few cases have been reported to make generalizations.

TRANSMISSIBLE VENEREAL TUMOR

Transmissible venereal tumor (TVT) was the first transplantable and transmissible tumor to be recorded. It is spread between dogs rather than arising from an individual dog's cells. The tumor even has a different number of chromosomes (often around fifty-nine) than do normal dog cells (seventy-eight). It is transmitted from dog to dog by sexual contact and direct contact associated with social behavior.

The tumors are often large cauliflower-like growths seen on the genitals or face. Metastasis is possible but not frequent. Tumors within the nasal cavity may result in nosebleeds (epistaxis) and sneezing. The diagnosis is made by biopsy, and various treatments have resulted in cures. Where feasible, the tumor should be completely excised. For localized areas where surgery would be difficult, radiation therapy is often effective. For systemic or metastatic disease, treatment is often with either doxorubicin HCl (Adriamycin) or vincristine sulfate until complete remission is achieved. This often requires about six weeks of therapy.

TRICHOEPITHELIOMA

Trichoepitheliomas are benign tumors of hair-producing cells and appear as round masses, usually on the back. They are frequently movable and unattached to underlying tissues. The skin overlying the mass may be hairless and ulcerated due to trauma. They are usually slow growing and benign and rarely spread or recur once removed.

TUMORAL CALCINOSIS

Tumoral calcinosis, or calcinosis circumscripta, is not a tumor in the classic sense of the word. It is a condition in which calcium is deposited in the skin, creating lumps that resemble tumors. The cause is currently not known.

The condition occurs predominantly in young, large-breed dogs; the German Shepherd Dog appears to be affected most often. It is seen as one or more nonpainful nodular lumps that may ulcerate and even discharge a white, pasty material. Most occur around the joints in the legs, but others may occur in the neck region, footpads, and even the mouth. Diagnosis is confirmed on the basis of biopsy. Since the underlying cause is a mystery, the best treatment at present is surgical removal of the lumps.

URTICARIA PIGMENTOSA

Urticaria pigmentosa is an accumulation of harmless mast cells, seen primarily in young dogs. The condition is fairly common in children, but it is relatively rare in dogs. It often looks like a small bump, but if the surface is briskly rubbed, the mast cells release their contents and hives form. It can be surgically removed if it is causing problems, but care must be taken to be gentle, since the original bump can be impossible to find if obscured by hives. Some cases of urticaria pigmentosa may regress on their own, since this is usually what happens in people.

9

BREED-RELATED SKIN DISORDERS

It has been known for years that certain skin problems are more common in some breeds than others, but to date the genetics of most of these conditions have not been well studied. There are many reasons for this, but to understand them, some basic knowledge of genetics is needed.

All puppies are the product of the genetic material of both parents. The sire contributes half of his genetic structure in his sperm, and the dam contributes half of her genetic structure in her ova (eggs). The split of genetic material is not random; for each individual trait there is a genetic component from each parent. Thus, if the puppy is a male (XY), it received its Y chromosome from the sire and its X chromosome from the dam. Female pups receive an X chromosome from each parent.

Genes are composed of DNA and are located on the chromosomes. In the dog, there are seventy-eight chromosomes; man has only forty-six. The chromosomes are arranged in pairs (thirty-nine pair in the dog), and of these, two are sex chromosomes; the rest are referred to as autosomes. Very few traits are carried on the sex chromosomes, so the vast majority are therefore described as being autosomal.

When a trait is completely controlled by one set of genes, it is called monogenic, but relatively few traits fit into this category. Of all the traits a pup may inherit from its parents, most are the product of many genes and are referred to as polygenic. This is also true in people. If a six-foot-tall man married a five-foot-tall woman and they had children, how tall would those children be? Height, weight, and most physical characteristics result from a complex interplay of many different genes, making this question impossible to answer with any real accuracy. What we often can say is that some traits seem to run in families, and we refer to this relationship as "familial" because we don't know the actual genetic basis. The same is true for dogs. Some traits run in different lines, and even though we may say some breeds are prone to certain diseases, it is really individual families or lines that are affected.

Two additional terms that are frequently used when discussing genetic problems are dominant and recessive. If a trait is recessive, then pups will only be affected if both parents carry that trait. If a trait is dominant, then pups can be affected if either parent carries the trait.

It must be kept in mind that not all skin diseases seen in the young are inherited; some may occur as a fluke of nature. On the other hand, it behooves us to recognize inherited conditions so that their incidence may be lessened by conscientious breeding. Those breeders and pet owners who would like to become involved with the study and data collection of different breed-related problems should contact:

Genodermatosis Research Foundation
1635 Grange Hall Road
Dayton, OH 45432
(513) 426-7060
This organization collects information
on breed-related skin disorders.

Genetic Disease Control
P.O. Box 222
Davis, CA 95617
(916) 756-6773
An open registry for all types of
inherited problems in animals,
including some skin problems.

Some conditions that are inherited (e.g., a tendency to develop allergies, defective immune systems, poor absorption or metabolism of essential nutrients) may not show up immediately in the newborn and may not manifest themselves until later in the animal's life. In the language of genetics, traits present at birth are referred to as congenital, while those that appear at some later date are called tardive.

In addition, certain animals have purposely been bred to have abnormal skin, such as the hairless breeds, for example, the Mexican Hairless, Abyssinian Dog, African Sand Dog, Chinese Crested Dog, Xoloitzcuintli, and the Turkish Naked Dog. Color mutant breeds include blue Dobermans,

Great Danes, Dachshunds, Whippets, and Standard Poodles. Dogs with excessively folded skin include Chinese Shar-peis and Pugs.

BREED PREDISPOSITIONS TO SKIN DISORDERS

Many conditions appear to be especially prominent in some breeds. Sometimes it is possible to identify the genetic basis of a problem, but in many cases we must be satisfied with identifying breeds that are at risk. As discussed above, it is really individual families at risk rather than whole breeds. These conditions are listed alphabetically, as are the breeds themselves.

Table 9.1. Breed Dispositions to Skin Disorders

Breed	Condition
Afghan Hound	Demodicosis
	Hypothyroidism
Airedale	Allergic inhalant dermatitis
	Growth hormone-responsive dermatosis
	Melanoma
	Seasonal alopecia
	Vascular nevi
Akita	Hypothyroidism
	Pemphigus foliaceus
	Sebaceous adenitis
	Uveodermatologic syndrome
Alaskan Malamute	Hypothyroidism
	Nasal solar dermatitis
	Zinc-responsive dermatosis
Basenji	Hypothyroidism
	Metabolic dermatosis
Basset Hound	Collagen nevi
	Combined immunodeficiency
	Interdigital pyoderma
	Sebaceous adenitis
	Sebaceous-gland tumors
	Seborrhea
Beagle	Allergic inhalant dermatitis
	Cutaneous asthenia
	Demodicosis
	Hemangiopericytoma
	Hepatoid-gland tumor
	Lipoma

Table 9.1. Continued

Breed	Condition
Beagle (cont.)	Lymphosarcoma
	Sebaceous-gland tumors
	Zinc-responsive dermatosis
Bearded Collie	Black hair follicular dysplasia
	Lupus erythematosus
Belgian Tervuren	Vitiligo
Bernese Mountain Dog	Hemangiosarcoma
	Malignant histiocytosis
Bichon Frise	Allergic inhalant dermatitis
Borzoi	Primary lymphedema
Boston Terrier	Allergic inhalant dermatitis
	Demodicosis
	Fibroma
	Hyperadrenocorticism
	Mast-cell tumor
	Melanoma
	Sebaceous-gland tumors
	Tail fold pyoderma
Boxer	Acne
	Callus (sternum)
	Coccidioidomycosis
	Cutaneous asthenia
	Demodicosis
	Dermoid sinus
	Fibroma
	Hemangioma
	Hemangiopericytoma
	Hemangiosarcoma
	Histiocytoma
	Hyperadrenocorticism
	Hypothyroidism
	Interdigital pyoderma
	Lymphosarcoma
	Mast-cell tumor
	Melanoma
	Seasonal alopecia
	Sertoli-cell tumor
	Squamous-cell carcinoma
Brittany	Hypothyroidism
	Liposarcoma
Bull Mastiff	Acne
Bull Terrier	Acrodermatitis
	Demodicosis
	Mast-cell tumor

Table 9.1. Continued

Breed	Condition
Bulldog	Acne
	Demodicosis
	Face fold pyoderma
	Hepatoid-gland tumor
	Hypothyroidism
	Interdigital pyoderma
	Mast-cell tumor
	Primary lymphedema
	Seasonal alopecia
	Sterile pyogranuloma
	Tail fold pyoderma
Cairn Terrier	Allergic inhalant dermatitis
	Vitamin A-responsive dermatosis
Chihuahua	Alopecia (congenital)
	Anal sacculitis
	Demodicosis
	Melanoma
	Sertoli-cell tumor
Chow Chow	Castration-responsive alopecia
	Color dilution alopecia
	Demodicosis
	Follicular dysplasia
	Growth hormone-responsive dermatosis
	Hypothyroidism
	Melanoma
	Sebaceous adenitis
	Tyrosinase deficiency
Cocker Spaniel	Allergic inhalant dermatitis
	Anal sacculitis
	Basal-cell tumor
	Canine cyclic hematopoiesis
	Cutaneous lymphoma
	Demodicosis
	Fibrosarcoma
	Hemangiopericytoma
	Hepatoid-gland tumors
	Histiocytoma
	Hypothyroidism
	Hypotrichosis
	Idiopathic seborrhea
	Lip fold pyoderma
	Lipoma

Table 9.1. Continued

Breed	Condition
Cocker Spaniel (cont.)	Lymphosarcoma
	Melanoma
	Nasodigital hyperkeratosis
	Papilloma
	Sebaceous-gland tumor
	Sweat-gland tumors
	Trichoepithelioma
	Vitamin A-responsive dermatosis
Collie	Adverse reactions to ivermectin
	Black hair follicular dysplasia
	Bullous pemphigoid
	Demodicosis
	Dermatomyositis
	Discoid lupus erythematosus
	Epidermolysis bullosa simplex
	Fibrous histiocytoma
	Gray Collie syndrome
	Intracutaneous cornifying epithelioma
	Nasal pyoderma
	Nasal solar dermatitis (?)
	Nodular panniculitis
	Pemphigus erythematosus
	Pemphigus foliaceus
	Pyotraumatic dermatitis
	Sebaceous adenitis
	Systemic lupus erythematosus
Dachshund	Acanthosis nigricans
	Black hair follicular dysplasia
	Callus pyoderma
	Color mutant alopecia
	Combined immunodeficiency
	Cutaneous asthenia
	Cutaneous vasculitis
	Demodicosis
	Ear margin dermatosis
	Hepatoid-gland tumors
	Histiocytoma hypothyroidism
	Hyperadrenocorticism
	Keratinization disorders
	Interdigital pyoderma
	Juvenile cellulitis
	Juvenile panniculitis
	Linear IgA dermatosis
	Lipoma
	Liposarcoma

Table 9.1. Continued

Breed	Condition
Dachshund (cont.)	Mast-cell tumor
	Pattern baldness
	Pinnal alopecia
	Sebaceous adenitis
	Sebaceous-gland tumor
	Sterile pyogranuloma
Dalmatian	Allergic inhalant dermatitis
	Dalmatian bronzing syndrome
	Demodicosis
	Sebaceous adenitis
Doberman Pinscher	Acne
	Acral lick dermatitis
	Adverse reaction to sulfa drugs
	Bullous pemphigoid
	Callus
	Coccidioidomycosis
	Color mutant alopecia
	Demodicosis
	Flank sucking
	Focal mucinosis
	Hypopigmentation of lips
	Hypothyroidism
	Ichthyosis
	Interdigital pododermatitis
	Lipoma
	Sebaceous adenitis
	Systemic lupus erythematosus
	Vitiligo
	Zinc-responsive dermatosis
Fox Terrier	Fibroma
	Hemangiopericytoma
	Juvenile panniculitis
	Mast-cell tumor
	Nodular panniculitis
	Schwannoma
German Shepherd Dog	Acral lick dermatitis
	Callus
	Collagen nevi
	Cutaneous asthenia
	Demodicosis
	Discoid lupus erythematosus
	Familial vasculopathy
	Furunculosis
	Hemangioma

Table 9.1. Continued

Breed	Condition
German Shepherd Dog (cont.)	Hemangiopericytoma
	Hemangiosarcoma
	Hepatoid-gland tumor
	Interdigital pyoderma
	Intracutaneous cornifying epithelioma
	Juvenile footpad disease
	Lymphosarcoma
	Nasal pyoderma
	Nasal solar dermatitis
	Nodular dermatofibrosis
	Perianal fistulae
	Pituitary dwarfism
	Primary lymphedema
	Pyotraumatic dermatitis
	Sebaceous adenitis
	Tumoral calcinosis
	Tyrosinemia
	Vitiligo
	Zinc-responsive dermatosis
Golden Retriever	Allergic inhalant dermatitis
	Collagen nevi
	Hypothyroidism
	Ichthyosis
	Juvenile cellulitis
	Lymphosarcoma
	Pyotraumatic dermatitis
	Sebaceous adenitis
	Uveodermatologic syndrome
Great Dane	Acne
	Acral lick dermatitis
	Callus
	Color mutant alopecia
	Demodicosis
	Dermoid cyst
	Histiocytoma
	Hypothyroidism
	Interdigital pyoderma
	Primary lymphedema
	Sterile pyogranuloma
	Tumoral calcinosis
	Zinc-responsive dermatosis
Greyhound	Color mutant alopecia
	Cutaneous asthenia
Irish Setter	Acral lick dermatitis
	Allergic inhalant dermatitis

Table 9.1. Continued

Breed	Condition
Irish Setter (cont.)	Callus
	Canine granulocytopathy syndrome
	Color mutant alopecia
	Hypothyroidism
	Keratinization disorders
	Melanoma
	Sebaceous adenitis (granulomatous)
	Uveodermatologic syndrome
Irish Wolfhound	Hypothyroidism
Karelian Bear Dog	Pituitary dwarf
Keeshond	Growth hormone-responsive dermatosis
	Intracutaneous cornifying epithelioma
	Woolly syndrome
Kerry Blue Terrier	Dermoid sinus
	Papilloma
	Pilomatrixoma
	Sebaceous-gland tumor
	Spiculosis
	Vascular nevi
Labrador Retriever	Acral lick dermatitis
	Allergic inhalant dermatitis
	Contact allergy (?)
	Focal mucinosis
	Infantile pustular dermatosis
	Interdigital pododermatitis
	Lipoma
	Mast-cell tumor
	Primary lymphedema
	Pyotraumatic dermatitis
	Sebaceous adenitis
	Vascular nevi
	Vitamin A-responsive dermatosis
Lhasa Apso	Allergic inhalant dermatitis
	Sebaceous adenitis
Malamute	Eosinophilic granuloma
	Hypothyroidism
	Woolly syndrome
	Zinc-responsive dermatosis
Mexican Hairless	Congenital alopecia
Newfoundland	Callus
	Hypothyroidism
	Sterile pyogranuloma

Table 9.1. Continued

Breed	Condition
Norwegian Elkhound	Intracutaneous cornifying epithelioma
	Sebaceous-gland tumor
	Squamous-cell carcinoma
Old English Sheepdog	Demodicosis
	Intracutaneous cornifying epithelioma
	Primary lymphedema
	Sebaceous adenitis
	Uveodermatologic syndrome
Papillon	Black hair follicular dysplasia
Pekingese	Face fold pyoderma
	Squamous-cell carcinoma
Pointer	Acral mutilation syndrome
	Callus
	Demodicosis
	Hereditary lupoid dermatosis (of German Shorthairs)
	Juvenile cellulitis
	Nasal pyoderma
Pomeranian	Canine cyclic hematopoiesis
	Hyperadrenocorticism
	Growth hormone-responsive dermatosis
	Sertoli-cell tumor
Poodle	Allergic inhalant dermatitis
	Anal licking
	Anal sacculitis
	Basal-cell tumor
	Color mutant alopecia
	Cutaneous T-cell-like lymphoma
	Growth hormone-responsive dermatosis
	Hyperadrenocorticism
	Hypothyroidism
	Hypotrichosis
	Ichthyosis
	Junctional epidermolysis bullosa
	Juvenile panniculitis
	Lipoma
	Nodular panniculitis
	Pilomatrixoma
	Primary lymphedema
	Sebaceous adenitis
	Sebaceous-gland nevi
	Sebaceous-gland tumor
	Sertoli-cell tumor
	Squamous-cell carcinoma
	Zinc-responsive dermatosis

Table 9.1. Continued

Breed	Condition
Portuguese Water Dog	Alopecia
Pug	Allergic inhalant dermatitis Demodicosis Face fold pyoderma Tail fold pyoderma
Rhodesian Ridgeback	Dermoid sinus
Rottweiler	Acne Hypothyroidism Interdigital pododermatitis
St. Bernard	Callus Cutaneous asthenia Lip fold pyoderma Pyotraumatic dermatitis Sterile pyogranuloma
Saluki	Color dilution alopecia
Samoyed	Hepatoid-gland tumor Nasal solar dermatitis Sebaceous adenitis (granulomatous) Uveodermatologic syndrome Zinc-responsive dermatosis
Schipperke	Black hair follicular dysplasia
Schnauzer	Acquired aurotrichia Adverse reaction to herbal shampoos Allergic inhalant dermatitis Cutaneous asthenia Hypothyroidism Schnauzer comedo syndrome Sertoli-cell tumor Subcorneal pustular dermatosis Vitamin A-responsive dermatosis
Scottish Terrier	Allergic inhalant dermatitis Lymphosarcoma Melanoma Sebaceous adenitis Squamous-cell carcinoma Vascular nevi
Shar-pei	Allergic inhalant dermatitis Body fold pyoderma Demodicosis Face fold pyoderma Focal mucinosis

Table 9.1. Continued

Breed	Condition
Shar-pei (cont.)	Folliculitis
	Food allergy/intolerance (?)
	Hypothyroidism
	IgA deficiency
	Infantile pustular dermatitis
	Interdigital pododermatitis
	Keratinization disorders
	Lip fold pyoderma
	Pemphigus foliaceus (?)
Shetland Sheepdog	Bullous pemphigoid (?)
	Castration-responsive alopecia
	Dermatomyositis
	Discoid lupus erythematosus
	Epidermolysis bullosa simplex (?)
	Focal mucinosis
	Histiocytoma
	Nasal solar dermatitis
	Pemphigus erythematosus (?)
	Sertoli-cell tumor
	Systemic lupus erythematosus
Shih Tzu	Allergic inhalant dermatitis
	Dermoid sinus
Siberian Husky	Discoid lupus erythematosus
	Eosinophilic granuloma
	Sertoli-cell tumor
	Uveodermatologic syndrome
	Woolly syndrome
	Zinc-responsive dermatosis
Springer Spaniel	Cutaneous asthenia
	Hemangiopericytoma
	Keratinization disorders
	Lichenoid-psoriasiform dermatitis
	Lip fold pyoderma
	Melanoma
	Sebaceous adenitis
Staffordshire Terrier	Demodicosis
	Mast-cell tumor
Viszla	Hypothyroidism
	Sebaceous adenitis
Weimaraner	Lipoma
	Mast-cell tumor
	Sebaceous adenitis
	T-cell immunodeficiency

Table 9.1. Continued

Breed	Condition
Welsh Corgi	Cutaneous asthenia
	Nasal solar dermatitis
West Highland Terrier	Allergic inhalant dermatitis
	Ichthyosis
	Keratinization disorders (epidermal dysplasia, seborrhea)
	Yeast dermatitis
Whippet	Color mutant alopecia
	Hypotrichosis
Yorkshire Terrier	Allergic inhalant dermatitis
	Color dilution alopecia
	Sertoli-cell tumor

The above list may seem daunting, but it must be remembered that all genetic risks are "relative" and are more correctly associated with lines and families than the breed in general. The existence of the following conditions does not mean that certain breeds as a whole are "tainted" by hereditary skin diseases.

SPECIFIC BREED-RELATED PROBLEMS

Acanthosis Nigricans

Acanthosis nigricans is a condition in which the skin of the underarm and groin areas becomes very thick and darkly pigmented. The suspected inherited disorder is almost exclusively limited to the Dachshund. The diagnosis is often incorrectly used for dogs with other skin problems, such as allergies, in which these areas are also affected and become darkened from the inflammation present in the skin.

In time, Dachshunds with acanthosis nigricans develop very thick, dark, and hairless skin on their whole underside and become quite greasy. Diagnosis should be carefully made on the basis of biopsy.

The treatment of true acanthosis nigricans is difficult, because the reason for it is unknown. The most conservative therapies combine using vitamin E (200 IU twice daily) with antiseborrheic shampoos that dissolve grease (e.g., selenium, tar, benzoyl peroxide). Topical corticosteroids are also used sometimes to help reduce inflammation, but long-term safety must be considered when selecting products. Also, a pineal gland extract, melatonin, has been used experimentally to counteract the darkening of the skin seen in this condition.

Color Plates for Chapter 2

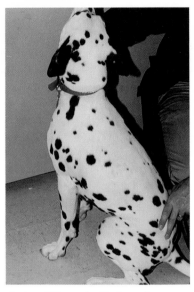

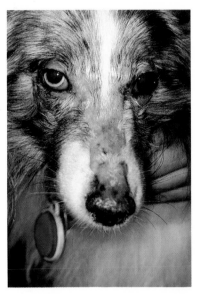

Color Plate 1. Dalmatian bronzing syndrome. This is a subtle, early change in the color of the haircoat on the back. From, Ackerman, L: *Practical Canine Dermatology,* American Veterinary Publications, 1989.

Color Plate 2. Dermatomyositis. A more severe case. Photo courtesy of Dr. T. Lewis.

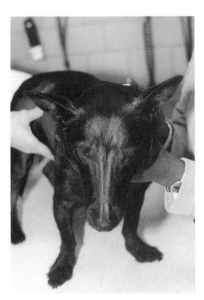

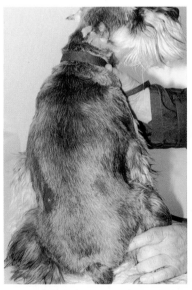

Color Plate 3. Follicular dysplasia. There is a loss of hair on the face as a result of the developmental defect of the hairs in this area.

Color Plate 4. Gilding syndrome (aurotrichia) in a Schnauzer.

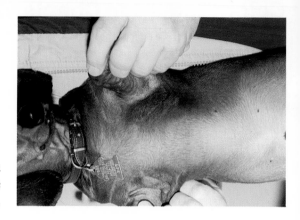

Color Plate 5. Acanthosis nigricans in a Dachshund. Note the darkening of the skin in the armpits.

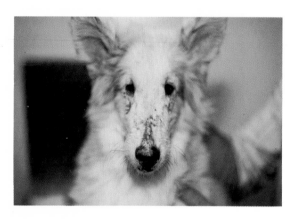

Color Plate 6. Dermatomyositis. A mild case in a pup. This condition can result in scarring, especially on the face.

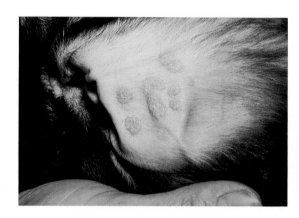

Color Plate 7. Lichenoid-psoriasiform dermatitis on the ear of a Springer Spaniel.

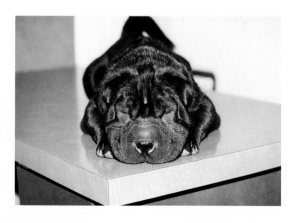

Color Plate 8. Mucinosis in a Chinese Shar-Pei. Photo courtesy of Dr. T. Lewis.

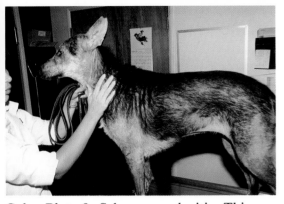

Color Plate 9. Sebaceous adenitis. This represents one manifestation of the disorder but there are several others. Photo courtesy of Dr. T. Lewis.

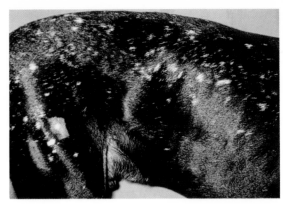

Color Plate 10. Vitiligo in a Doberman Pinscher.

Color Plates for Chapter 3

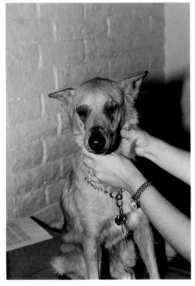

Color Plate 11. Mild symptoms of inhalant allergies. Note the dark patches around the eyes.

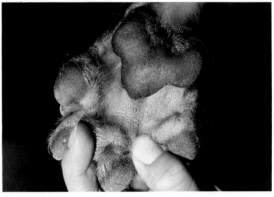

Color Plate 12. Most dogs with inhalant allergies lick their feet because of the inflammation. Photo courtesy of Dr. T. Lewis.

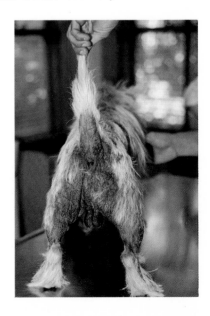

Color Plate 13. More severe changes associated with long-standing and poorly controlled allergies.

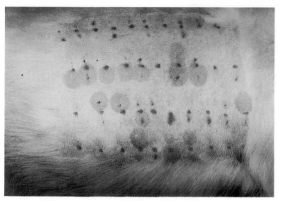

Color Plate 14. Intradermal allergy testing. Dots (red) are used to mark the location of injected allergens. Positive reactions come up as hives.

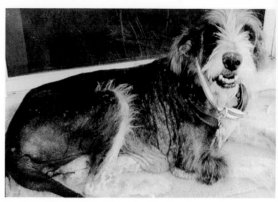

Color Plate 15. Food allergy in a dog. Photo courtesy of Dr. T. Lewis.

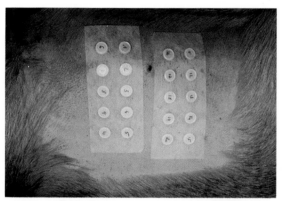

Color Plate 16. Complicated "patch test," used to diagnose contact allergies in the dog. Photo by Dr. Thiery Olivry—provided by Dr. T. Lewis.

Color Plates for Chapter 4

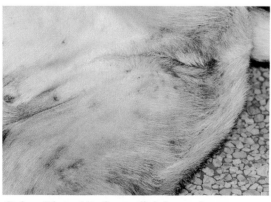

Color Plate 17. Superficial pyoderma (impetigo) in a puppy.

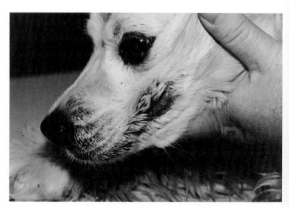

Color Plate 18. Lip fold pyoderma.

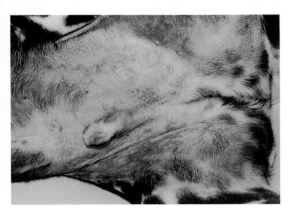

Color Plate 19. Bacterial infection of the hair follicles (folliculitis). From, Ackerman, L.: *Practical Canine Dermatology,* American Veterinary Publications, 1989.

Color Plate 20. Folliculitis on the topline of a dog. Because of the round appearance of the infection, it is often mistaken for "ringworm." From, Ackerman, L.: *Practical Canine Dermatology,* American Veterinary Publications, 1989.

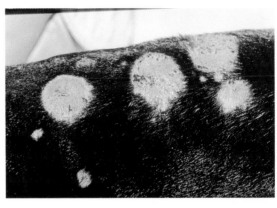

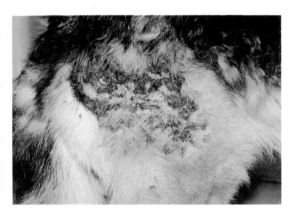

Color Plate 21. Deep pyoderma in a German Shepherd Dog. From, Ackerman, L.: *Practical Canine Dermatology,* American Veterinary Publications, 1989.

Color Plate 22. Perianal pyoderma (perianal fistulae) in a German Shepherd Dog. From, Ackerman, L.: *Practical Canine Dermatology,* American Veterinary Publications, 1989.

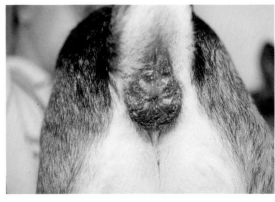

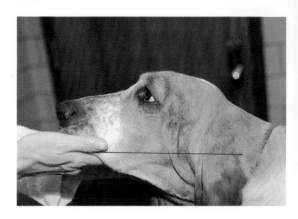

Color Plate 23. A very mild case of dermatophytosis.

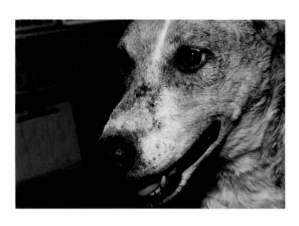

Color Plate 24. More aggressive case of dermatophytosis. Photo courtesy of Dr. T. Lewis.

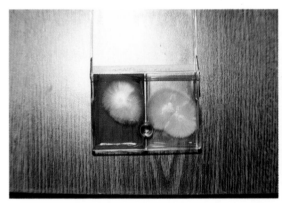

Color Plate 25. Dermatophyte Test Medium (DTM) is used to help diagnose dermatophytosis. Most ringworm fungi grow as white fluffy colonies and change the color of the medium from yellow to red.

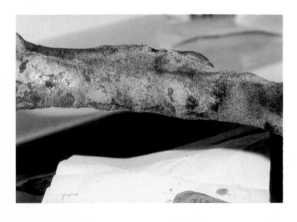

Color Plate 26. Intermediate and deep fungal infections can be very severe. This dog has sporotrichosis.

Color Plates for Chapter 5

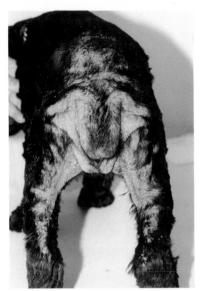

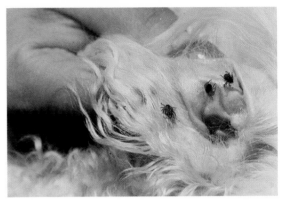

Color Plate 28. The ears make an excellent hiding place for ticks. Photo courtesy of Dr. T. Lewis.

Color Plate 27. Long-standing flea bite dermatitis. Note the hair loss, scaling, and thickening of the skin. From, Ackerman, L.: *Practical Canine Dermatology,* American Veterinary Publications, 1989.

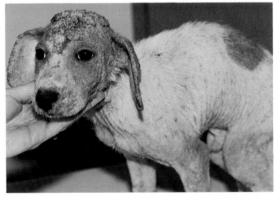

Color Plate 29. Demodectic mange in a puppy.

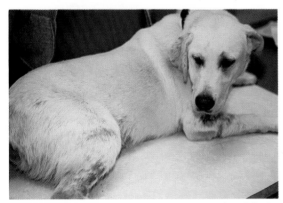

Color Plate 30. Sarcoptic mange (scabies) is exceptionally itchy and dogs can do severe damage to the skin by repeated chewing.

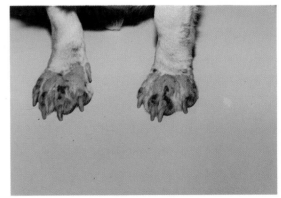

Color Plate 31. Pelodera dermatitis is caused by worms that penetrate the skin. Clinically, it is very similar to hookworm dermatitis.

Color Plates for Chapter 6

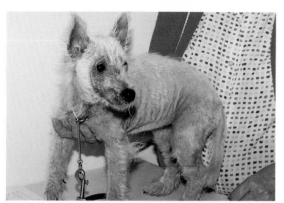

Color Plate 32. Epidermal dysplasia in a young West Highland White Terrier.

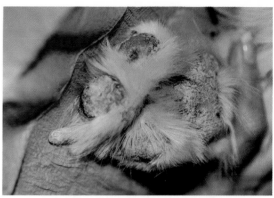

Color Plate 33. Hyperkeratotic footpads in a dog with zinc-responsive dermatitis.

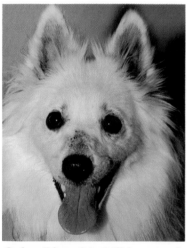

Color Plate 34. Mild case of zinc-responsive dermatitis. Note the scaling on the bridge of the nose. From, Ackerman, L.: *Practical Canine Dermatology,* American Veterinary Publications, 1989.

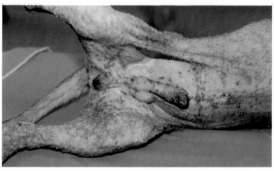

Color Plate 35. Generic dog food disease. From, Ackerman, L.: *Practical Canine Dermatology,* American Veterinary Publications, 1989.

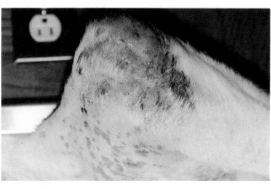

Color Plate 36. Inflamed callus on the elbow of a dog.

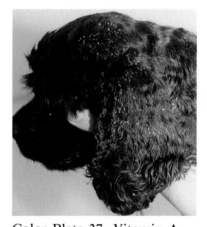

Color Plate 37. Vitamin A-responsive dermatosis in a Cocker Spaniel. Note the scale which clings to the hair. From, Ackerman, L.: *Practical Canine Derma-tology,* American Veterinary Publications, 1989.

Color Plates for Chapter 7

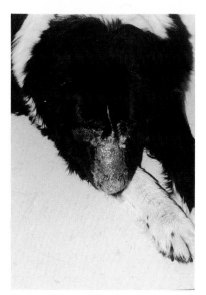

Color Plate 38. Skin changes associated with systemic lupus erythematosus.

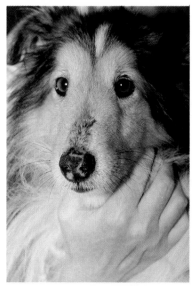

Color Plate 39. Cutaneous (discoid) lupus erythematosus. Note the loss of pigment on the inner aspects of the nose.

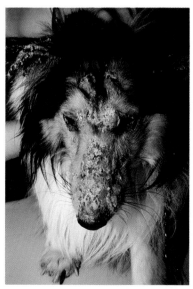

Color Plate 40. Pemphigus foliaceus with severe facial crusting. From, Ackerman, L.: *Practical Canine Dermatology,* American Veterinary Publications, 1989.

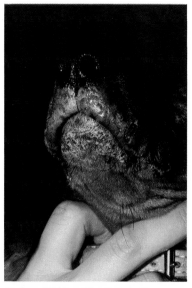

Color Plate 41. Juvenile cellulitis in a puppy.

Color Plate 42. Uveodermatological (VKH) syndrome in an Akita. There is loss of pigment around the lips and an immune-mediated eye disease. From, Ackerman, L.: *Practical Canine Dermatology,* American Veterinary Publications, 1989.

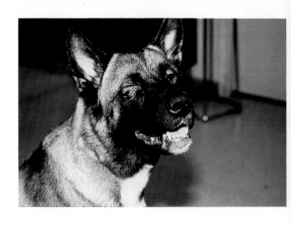

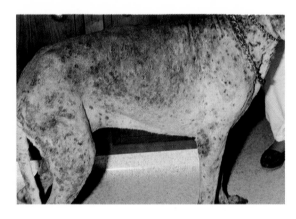

Color Plate 43. Generalized vasculitis, presenting as pinpoint scabs.

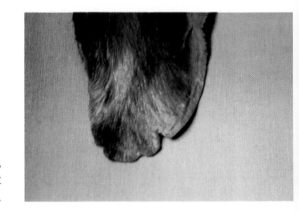

Color Plate 44. Vasculitis of the ear tips, which results in notching. This is most commonly seen in the Dachshund.

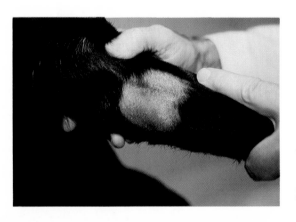

Color Plate 45. Alopecia areata on the front leg of a dog. From, Ackerman, L.: *Practical Canine Dermatology,* American Veterinary Publications, 1989.

Color Plates for Chapter 8

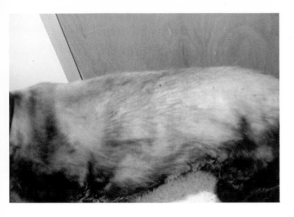

Color Plate 46. Hypothyroidism in an Irish Setter. There is symmetrical hair loss on the back. From, Ackerman, L.: *Practical Canine Dermatology,* American Veterinary Publications, 1989.

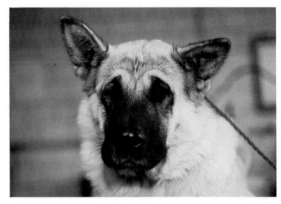

Color Plate 47. "Tragic expression" associated with hypothyroidism.

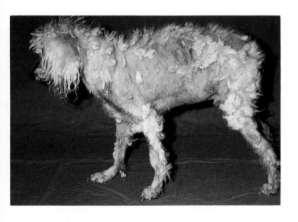

Color Plate 48. Cushing's syndrome in advanced stages.

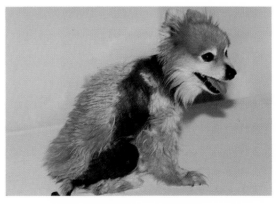

Color Plate 49. Growth hormone-responsive dermatosis.

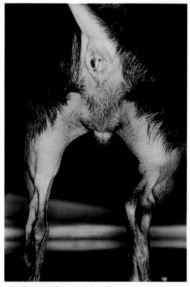

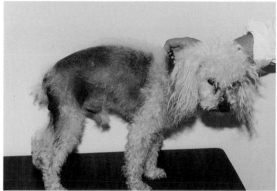

Color Plate 51. Hair loss associated with male feminizing syndrome.

Color Plate 50. Suspected hypoestrogenism.

Color Plates for Chapter 9

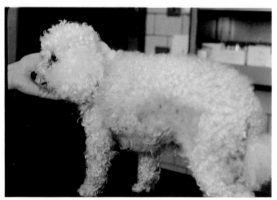

Color Plate 52. Cutaneous T-cell lymphoma (mycosis fungoides) is often difficult to diagnose initially because it doesn't look like a cancer. The redness and scaling may be confused with allergies or keratinization disorders.

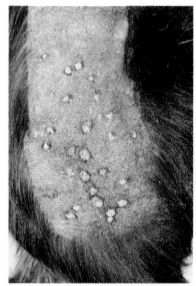

Color Plate 53. Squamous papillomas (warts). These are not caused by viruses.

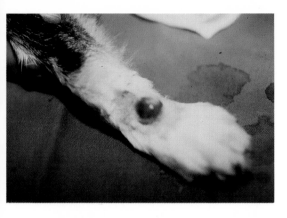

Color Plate 54. Large cyst on the foot of a dog.

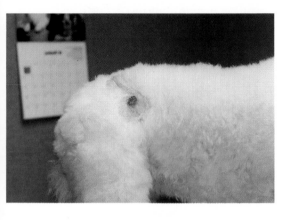

Color Plate 55. A granulomatous disorder in a dog caused by a reaction to vaccination.

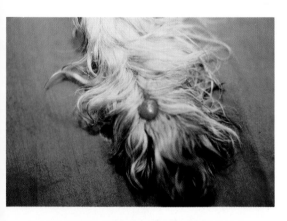

Color Plate 56. Histiocytoma. From, Ackerman, L.: *Practical Canine Dermatology,* American Veterinary Publications, 1989.

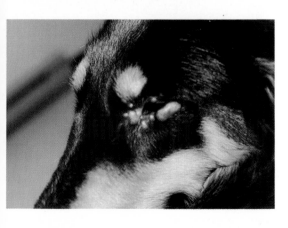

Color Plate 57. Nodular fasciitis (fibrous histiocytoma) is usually found around the eyes and lips.

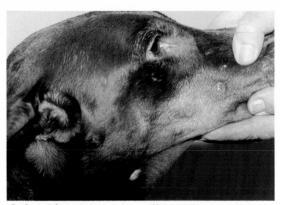

Color Plate 58. Mast-cell tumors on the head and neck of a Doberman Pinscher.

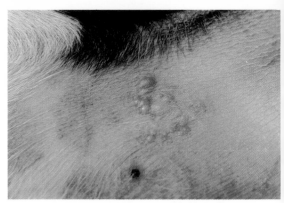

Color Plate 59. Urticaria pigmentosa, the harmless accumulation of mast cells in the skin.

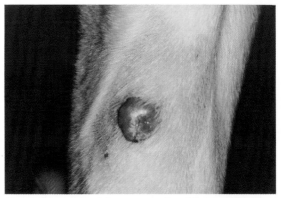

Color Plate 60. Sebaceous-gland hyperplasia, frequently mistaken for "warts." These are by far more common than are papillomas. Photo courtesy of Dr. T. Lewis.

Color Plates for Chapter 10

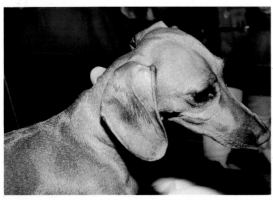

Color Plate 61. Pinnal alopecia on a Dachshund. Photo courtesy of Dr. T. Lewis.

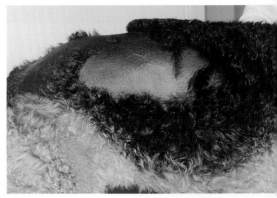

Color Plate 62. Seasonal (periodic) alopecia.

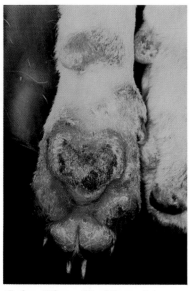

Color Plate 63. Hyperkeratotic footpads. Photo courtesy of Dr. T. Lewis.

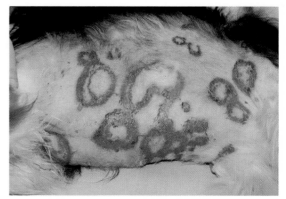

Color Plate 64. Superficial necrolytic dermatitis resulting from internal diseases. From, Ackerman, L.: *Practical Canine Dermatology,* American Veterinary Publications, 1989.

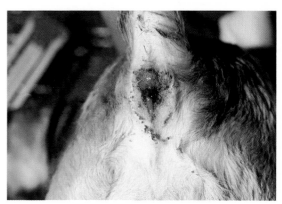

Color Plate 65. Anal sac abscess.

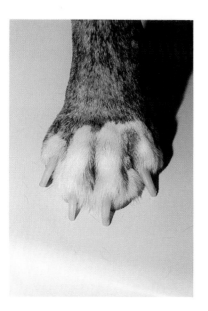

Color Plate 66. Interdigital dermatitis, in this case due to sterile pyogranuloma.

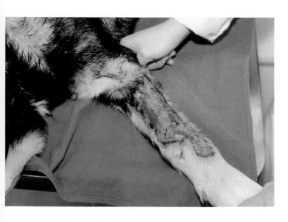

Color Plate 67. Acral lick dermatitis with significant damage to the skin of the leg. From, Ackerman, L.: *Practical Canine Dermatology,* American Veterinary Publications, 1989.

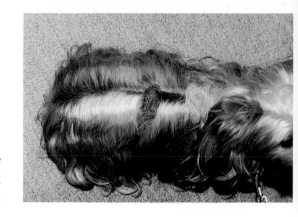

Color Plate 68. A burn is usually only obvious days later when it forms a black "eschar" and hair loss is evident.

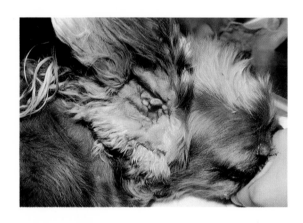

Color Plate 69. Ceruminous otitis in a Cocker Spaniel with a keratinization disorder. Photo courtesy of Dr. T. Lewis.

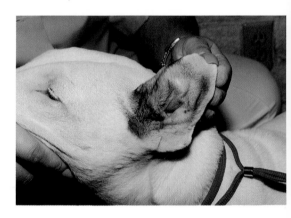

Color Plate 70. Inflammation of the ear flaps, associated in this case with inhalant allergies. Photo courtesy of Dr. T. Lewis.

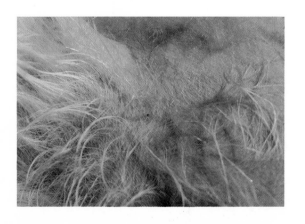

Color Plate 71. Area of traction alopecia, caused by incorrect placement of elastics, bows, and other constrictive devices. Photo courtesy of Dr. T. Lewis.

Acanthosis nigricans in people is quite different and usually suggests some form of internal cancer, but this is not the case in dogs. Therefore, safety must always be considered when evaluating therapies.

Acral Mutilation Syndrome

Acral mutilation syndrome is a bizarre condition reported in German Shorthaired Pointer and English Pointer pups. It is probably inherited as an autosomal recessive trait, which means that the pups must inherit an abnormal gene from both parents to be affected. The problem is not in the skin itself, but rather in the nerves that supply the legs. Affected animals lose pain sensation in their toes at about 3–5 months of age, and eventually they start chewing at their feet, mutilating them. Chewing at the feet is common in allergies and other conditions, but not to the point of mutilation.

This rare condition can be diagnosed by specific tests (electromyography), but no cure has been found. Obviously, these dogs should not be bred, nor should their parents have further offspring.

Acrodermatitis

Acrodermatitis is a skin disorder seen as a part of a fatal condition in Bull Terriers and is inherited as an autosomal recessive trait. Affected pups do not grow properly and develop infections of their feet and face, as well as diarrhea, pneumonia, and abnormal behavior. They generally die before they're a year and a half old. These pups often have a lighter coloring than normal littermates, which becomes accentuated with time. Pups that are only mildly affected may survive longer.

The reason these pups die is unknown, but many theories have been proposed, including a relative zinc imbalance or an abnormal thymus gland (important for the immune system).

Treatment to date has been unsuccessful in most cases. These dogs do not respond to zinc supplementation and eventually die because of overwhelming infection, usually pneumonia. Recently, however, some successful treatment has been reported with ketoconazole, a drug used to treat fungal infections. Etretinate, a synthetic vitamin A derivative, is also being evaluated and may be of some benefit. It is important that neither parent of pups with acrodermatitis be used in further breedings.

Canine Cyclic Hematopoiesis (Gray Collie Syndrome)

Some Collie pups born with a silver-gray haircoat may be smaller and weaker than their normal littermates and may have a light-colored nose. This condition appears to be transmitted as an autosomal recessive trait. By the age of 8–12 weeks, affected dogs start to develop bizarre symptoms such as fever, diarrhea, eye infections, painful joints (arthralgia), and abnormalities of their white blood cells. This syndrome has also now been reported in Pomeranians and Cocker Spaniels, so the descriptive term is preferred to Gray Collie syndrome.

When blood samples are collected daily over a two-week period, the neutrophils, a type of white blood cell, are seen to fluctuate from high to low over an 11–14-day cycle. When the neutrophils are at their lowest point, these pups are very susceptible to overwhelming infection; they usually die during these periods.

Diagnosis can be confirmed by sequential blood counts over a fourteen-day period. Therapy is invariably unsuccessful. However, treatment can be attempted with daily endotoxin (a bacterial toxin) or lithium. Bone marrow transplants have also been used experimentally to correct the blood cell defect. These are heroic efforts and not invariably successful. Parents and littermates should not be used for breeding.

Color Dilution Alopecia

Color dilution alopecia, also known as color mutant alopecia, describes a patchy, poor haircoat that can develop in animals bred for unusual hair color. Dogs that most often have this problem include blue Doberman Pinschers, Great Danes, Dachshunds, Whippets, Chow Chows, Italian Greyhounds, and Standard Poodles. Red Doberman Pinschers and fawn Irish Setters may have milder forms of the disorder. The condition has also been found in gray-blue Yorkshire Terriers, tricolor Salukis, and a blue-and-white mixed-breed dog. It is supposed that an abnormal gene (allele) on the d (dilution) locus is responsible for the problem. These animals are born with normal coats but later suffer from hair loss, dry skin, and bacterial infections. If one looks closely, the skin disease is confined only to unusually colored hairs.

Color dilution alopecia can be suspected just by looking at the dog, but confirmation of the diagnosis requires biopsy or examining plucked hairs microscopically. Because the hair follicles actually develop abnormally, there is no cure for this disorder. Hair does not regrow with thyroid medication or zinc supplementation. However, medicated shampoos can remove the prominent scale that forms on the skin surface, and emollients and moisturizers can help the dry skin. This therapy should be considered lifelong, and affected animals should not be used for breeding. If the abnormal allele on the d (dilution) locus is identified, a prevention program should be possible.

Cutaneous Asthenia

Cutaneous asthenia (Ehlers-Danlos syndrome) is a biochemical disorder where a low reserve of collagen causes the skin to be overly fragile and stretchable. Collagen is the fibrous connective tissue of the body. Animals with this problem are the rubber men of the dog world. When the skin of affected dogs is pulled, it can stretch to the point of tearing. Affected breeds include the Beagle, Dachshund, Boxer, St. Bernard, German Shepherd Dog, English Springer Spaniel, Greyhound, Schnauzer, and mongrels. The genetic nature of the condition is complex, but there is much evidence to suggest that it is a dominant trait.

The condition is usually easily diagnosed, but if there is any question, a series of measurements can be taken that will indicate the extent of the skin's stretchability. Biopsies are sometimes helpful but are not diagnostic in all cases.

There is no specific treatment for cutaneous asthenia because there is no method to overcome the inherited collagen defect. Large doses of vitamin C (collagen can't be manufactured without vitamin C) may be given as a supportive treatment but this will not cure the biochemical problem. These animals should definitely not be bred. Further, it is usually not safe for them to undergo surgery, even neutering.

Dalmatian Bronzing Syndrome

Dalmatian bronzing syndrome likely reflects an inherited defect in the metabolism of uric acid, accumulation of which can result in gout in people. Dalmatians with this defect form urinary "stones," suffer from recurrent urinary tract infections and skin infections, and may develop a coat that looks motheaten and which may even change color to a bronze hue (hence the name), especially along the back. The reason for this color change has not been determined.

The diagnosis can be suspected based on breed, symptoms, and biopsy findings, but blood tests for uric acid and the analysis of urine samples should also be done. Since most Dalmatians have higher uric acid levels than other breeds, these levels must be especially high to confirm a diagnosis.

The condition can easily be controlled by limiting the amount of specific proteins (purines) in the diet and/or by treating with drugs that lower blood uric acid levels (allopurinol). Commercial prescription diets are available from veterinarians (Hill's u/d), or recipes for diets are available that substitute eggs and vegetables for meats (which are particularly high in purines).

Dermatomyositis

Dermatomyositis is seen mostly in Collies, Shetland Sheepdogs, and their crosses, but has also been reported in an Australian Cattle Dog, Basset

Hound, and Pembroke Welsh Collie. It is an inflammatory disease of the skin, muscle, and sometimes, blood vessels. The condition is presumed to be inherited as an autosomal dominant trait, which means that only one parent needs to be affected to pass on the defect to the offspring. It has recently been proposed that an infectious agent (likely a virus) may actually instigate disease in genetically-prone pups. It is thought that this might then trigger an immune-mediated reaction similar to lupus erythematosus. The current theory is that pups that are genetically susceptible to dermatomyositis experience disease episodes only after being triggered by a viral infection. They then mount an immune-mediated reaction (similar to lupus) that causes the clinical signs (symptoms) that are seen.

Affected animals first begin to show signs of the condition at about 12 weeks of age. These may look like scrapes on the face, ears, elbows, hocks, and other friction points. The tip of the tail may also lose its hair. In later stages, there may be muscle wasting, especially on the top of the head (temporalis muscles) and over the hindquarters.

The condition is inherited as an autosomal dominant trait with variable expressivity. This means that if one parent is affected, most of the pups will be affected. This is an important consideration, since parents may only be mildly affected themselves but should be closely scrutinized if they produce affected young. Naturally, they should also not be bred again.

There is no blood test to identify carriers, and not enough data have been collected to permit pedigree analysis to select good breeding stock. Most cases are diagnosed on the basis of the history, clinical signs, electromyography, and biopsy. Well-chosen biopsies often reveal characteristic changes in the skin, and electromyographic (EMG) studies may show abnormalities in the muscles as well.

Therapy is only symptomatic. Pentoxifylline (Trental) is being evaluated experimentally for the management of severe cases, but optimal doses have not yet been established. Both vitamin E and corticosteroids have been used to relieve scaling and scarring, but neither will cure the condition. The disease usually determines its own path around the time of puberty, when some animals deteriorate further or recover spontaneously. Recovered animals should definitely not be bred, since offspring will undoubtedly be affected, at least to some extent.

Dermoid Sinus

A dermoid sinus is an abnormal congenital tract that connects the skin surface with the underlying spine. The tract is lined with skin and therefore eventually fills with dead skin, sebum, and bacteria, resulting in infection. Though the condition is most common on Rhodesian Ridgebacks, it has also been reported in the Boxer and Shih Tzu.

The diagnosis is usually confirmed by injecting dye into the tract and showing by x-rays that the channel has deep attachments. Surgical removal of the entire tract is the best treatment, and the affected animal usually recovers completely. These dogs should not be used for breeding.

Familial Benign Pemphigus

Also called Hailey-Hailey disease, this problem has recently been reported in English Setter puppies. Despite the name, the condition is not related to immune-mediated pemphigus. The condition starts within the first few months of age and small bumps enlarge into hairless areas with associated crusting. Diagnosis is by biopsy. No treatments are available. This is an autosomal dominant form of inheritance with variable expressivity presumed.

Familial Vasculopathy

This is a recently described disorder seen in young German Shepherd Dogs. These dogs have problems by 6–8 weeks of age, including lethargy, fever, and joint swelling. There is swelling of the nose, crusting and ulceration of ear margins and tail tip, and swelling and ulceration of the footpads. It is presumed, but not proven, that this represents some impairment of immune responsiveness. The condition often worsens following vaccination. Diagnosis is confirmed by biopsy. No medications have been reported to be helpful, but the condition may spontaneously improve.

Follicular Dysplasia

The term follicular dysplasia refers to a collection of disorders in which hair follicles that are normal at birth later become abnormal and stop producing hair. The condition is seen most commonly in animals less than a year old.

A breed-related dysplasia, in which guard hairs are shed and not replaced, appears to occur in the Siberian Husky. Once the guard hairs are gone, the undercoat takes on a rusty hue, and some of it may also be lost.

Black hair follicular dysplasia is seen in dogs with at least some black haircoat. Although affected dogs are normal at birth, they later begin to lose only black hairs in certain areas. The condition has been reported in both mongrels and purebreds, including the Dachshund, Papillon, Bearded Collie, and Schipperke. Although the exact mode of inheritance has not been established, when two affected individuals are bred, most of the offspring are affected by 4 weeks of age.

There are no blood tests to confirm the diagnosis of follicular dysplasia, and hormonal tests are invariably normal. Biopsies are the only way to verify the stage of growth of the follicles and any abnormalities they may have.

While there is no cure for follicular dysplasia, and dogs that have it should not be used for breeding, the condition does not affect a dog's general health.

Acquired Aurotrichia

Acquired aurotrichia, or gilding syndrome, is a condition that has recently been reported in Miniature Schnauzers in which their coat color changes from normal to a golden hue, especially along the topline. Most affected dogs are fairly young—generally about two and a half—when the disorder is detected. Diagnosis can be made visually, but confirmation requires a biopsy.

In a biopsied sample from an affected dog, there is a loss of pigment noted in the guard hairs, and the undercoat appears relatively atrophied. The pigment is not entirely absent, just lessened, and about half of all affected dogs eventually regain their normal color without medical intervention. The condition is seen equally in males and females, and no hormonal abnormalities have been detected to explain it. It may be diet related, or it may be a genetic disorder of pigmentation, although a pattern of inheritance has not been suggested.

Dogs with acquired aurotrichia should not be bred, but they are unlikely to suffer from any medical problems as a result of this condition.

Hypotrichosis

Congenital hypotrichosis (hairlessness from birth) is a rare defect reported in the Cocker Spaniel, Belgian Shepherd, Toy Poodle, Whippet, Bichon Frise, Basset Hound, Labrador Retriever, and Beagle. It is not known whether these breeds are affected by the same or different underlying disorders.

Diagnosis is usually not a problem, as the absence of hair is readily apparent. Biopsies of affected areas usually show a normal epidermis but no normal follicles present from which to grow hair. Since new follicles do not develop after birth, treatment is invariably unsuccessful.

Ichthyosis

In ichthyosis, the surface of the skin is covered by a thick, tenacious scale. The condition is rare but has been documented in West Highland White Terriers, Golden Retrievers, Cavalier King Charles Spaniels, Doberman Pinschers, Standard Poodles, and in a terrier mix. It is uncertain if all of these cases actually represent the same defect.

Diagnosis can usually be strongly suspected from clinical signs and biopsies, but treatment is intensive and difficult. Strong antiseborrheic products, including sulfur and/or tar shampoos, are helpful, as are lactic acid and urea products available from drugstores. Some of the newer vitamin A derivatives, such as retinoids and especially etretinate, may prove helpful in managing this condition. Even intense treatment, however, will only mask the disorder. As with all hereditary defects, treatment may improve the condition but does not offer a cure.

Lentigo

Lentigo (lentiginosis profusa) is a rare condition found most often in the Pug. Affected dogs have black spots on the skin caused by a localized increase in pigmentation. The trait that leads to lentigo may be autosomal dominant, but studies to prove that have not yet been done. Dogs with the condition remain healthy but cannot be shown. To date, no cases in the dog have later turned into malignant cancers such as melanoma. There is no practical therapy, although certain procedures to remove the spots (dermabrasion and electrodesiccation) have been used in people.

Lichenoid-Psoriasiform Dermatitis

Lichenoid-psoriasiform dermatitis is a harmless condition sometimes found in Springer Spaniels. Affected dogs develop bumps or wart-like projections on the inner flaps of the ears and occasionally on the abdomen. These areas may appear red and scaly, but they don't cause any real problems and are rarely itchy. Most dogs are fairly young (less than 3 years) when first affected. The condition may wax and wane but never clears entirely and doesn't respond to any treatments. Occasionally treatment is attempted with corticosteroids or vitamin A derivatives, but these rarely offer any real benefit. Treatment should not be excessive, since this condition does not affect the health of these otherwise normal dogs.

Lupoid Dermatosis

Hereditary lupoid dermatosis is a recently described skin problem seen most commonly in German Shorthaired Pointers. Most affected pups are 5 to 7 months of age (range is 4 months to 4 years) and develop thickening of the skin and scaling, which tends to begin on the head and back before becoming generalized. The most commonly affected areas are the head, hocks, and scrotum. The condition can also result in fragmentation and sloughing of the nails.

The diagnosis is made by biopsy and the name is derived from the finding that biopsies share some similarities with lupus erythematosus. The usual treatment has been aimed at controlling inflammation and prednisone and combinations of niacinamide and tetracycline have been advocated.

Mucinosis

Mucinosis is a somewhat rare and confusing condition in which the supporting network under the skin is replaced in areas by mucin, which is a secretion with the texture of mucus. This results in the presence of bumps and lumps in the skin. Breeds at greatest risk are the Chinese Shar-pei and Doberman Pinscher, but Shetland Sheepdogs and Labrador Retrievers have also been affected. Females may be more prone than males to developing mucinosis.

Diagnosis can only be confirmed by biopsy. It is assumed that mucinosis in the Chinese Shar-pei is inherited, and in fact, all Chinese Shar-peis have more mucin (mostly hyaluronic acid) in their skin than other dogs, which likely accounts, to some degree, for their wrinkles. Other breeds should be screened for underlying problems that might account for the mucin accumulation, including hypothyroidism, mucopolysaccharidosis, lupus erythematosus, dermatomyositis, scleroderma, and eosinophilic granuloma.

There is no need to treat dogs with mucinosis since their general health remains unaffected. It would be wise, however, not to use these dogs in any breeding program.

Nodular Dermatofibrosis

Nodular dermatofibrosis refers to a condition that occurs in adult German Shepherd Dogs in which they develop lumps, usually on their legs. The condition is important, not because of the lumps themselves, but because they are often associated with internal cancers affecting the kidneys and sometimes the uterus. These lumps are therefore an important "marker" that indicate that the dog should be carefully screened for cancer.

Diagnosis is made by biopsy of the lumps, and a good pathologist with expertise in skin problems should be able to confirm suspicions. A positive diagnosis means that the dog should be carefully checked for a specific cancer (cystadenocarcinoma) of the kidney. If only one kidney is affected and the cancer has not spread, surgical removal of that kidney may provide a cure. The skin lumps need not be removed.

It appears that nodular dermatofibrosis and the underlying problems associated with it are hereditary. The mode of inheritance is probably autosomal dominant. Unfortunately, the disease will be difficult to eliminate by breeding programs, because affected dogs do not show disease until later in life, after they may have produced offspring.

Sebaceous Adenitis

Sebaceous adenitis, also known as periappendageal dermatitis, is a recently discovered problem in which there is inflammatory damage of the hair follicles and the sebaceous glands that supply them. It is most commonly seen in the Standard Poodle but has also been reported in many other breeds, including the Vizsla, Samoyed, Irish Setter, Akita, Collie, Golden Retriever, Old English Sheepdog, Doberman Pinscher, Springer Spaniel, Basset Hound, Scottish Terrier, German Shepherd Dog, Miniature Poodle, Miniature Pinscher, Chow Chow, Weimaraner, Lhasa Apso, Dalmatian, Dachshund, and some mixed breeds.

Most animals are in young adulthood when they first develop flaking of the skin and then a loss of hair. In general, the condition is not itchy or irritating unless the dogs have managed to develop infection in these sites. Other than these changes, the dogs appear to remain in good health.

It may very well be that different breeds actually have different disorders, but at present the term sebaceous adenitis is used as a general description rather than a diagnosis until the disease is better understood. A new classification system for sebaceous adenitis divides most long-haired breeds (e.g., Standard Poodle, Old English Sheepdog, Samoyed, Akita) into Type I, in which the condition progresses rapidly and responds to symptomatic therapy only. Type II is seen in the Viszla and other short-coated breeds; it progresses slowly and responds best to retinoids and cyclosporine.

Proper diagnosis requires biopsies, and they should be sent to veterinary pathololgists with expertise in skin disorders. In the Standard Poodle, normal-appearing carriers can sometimes even be detected by early biopsies. Animals that appear normal but that have more than two hair follicles affected out of two 6mm punch biopsies are classified as subclinical and should not be used for breeding. These biopsies are usually taken from the topline between the head and the shoulder blades. For breeds other than the Standard Poodle, two 6mm biopsies should be taken from affected areas early in the course of the disorder, when changes are most likely to be evident.

Early cases are often treated with corticosteroids, which may or may not help. Some preliminary work has been done with isotretinoin, a synthetic form of vitamin A used in the treatment of acne. This is more effective in the Viszla and Standard Poodle than in other breeds. Etretinate, another form of synthetic vitamin A, is somewhat more effective in the Akita, which generally responds poorly to all forms of therapy. Antibiotics are usually also helpful for Akitas because they tend to have more bacterial complications than the other breeds. Using essential fatty acid supplements in all cases is a good idea, because they are mildly anti-inflammatory and have few or no side effects.

Topical treatment is important with sebaceous adenitis, because the skin becomes very dry and scaly. This means frequent shampooing with products that help remove surface scale (e.g., tar, sulfur, salicylic acid, selenium sulfide) and moisturizing the skin with rinses of 50% propylene glycol and various other moisturizers, emollients, and humectants. Hot oil treatments or human products that contain lactic acid or urea may be helpful but require intensive owner commitment.

Spiculosis

Spiculosis refers to a hair shaft disorder in Kerry Blue Terriers. In one report, affected dogs were 6–30 months old when first affected, and all three were male. Hairs on the face, trunk, and extremities were brittle and thick, and had nodules present that were later referred to as spicules. The spicules were so named because of their spiny appearance under the microscope. These abnormal hairs may result from fusion of the primary and secondary hairshafts, but this has not been determined. Spiculosis does not appear to affect a dog's health, and no treatment is needed other than clipping the affected hairs.

Vitiligo

Vitiligo describes a patchy loss of pigment that may be inherited or acquired. In general it refers to white patches that occur on the surface of the skin. Whitening of the hairs is more correctly referred to as leukotrichia and graying of the hairs as poliosis. Loss of pigment can be but is not necessarily inherited. A heritable form of vitiligo may be seen in Belgian Tervurens, Labrador Retrievers, Rottweilers, and Doberman Pinschers (Dudley nose), though the actual heritability has not been confirmed. A similar loss of pigment in Chow Chows is due to an inherited deficiency of tyrosinase, an enzyme important in pigment production. Leukotrichia has been reported in Labrador Retrievers, which may start to show whitening of the hairs on the face, back, and legs by 8 weeks of age. In the cases that have been studied, the condition resolved on its own by the time the dogs were 14 weeks old, with no need for treatment.

Loss of pigment can also occur with a number of nongenetic disorders, including autoimmune disorders (e.g., autoimmune vitiligo, lupus erythematosus, Vogt-Koyanagi-Harada-like syndrome), some cancers (e.g., melanoma, cutaneous T-cell lymphoma), and as a consequence of inflammatory damage.

Since it is important to differentiate nonharmful inherited problems from potentially dangerous nongenetic problems, biopsies and blood tests should be performed on all suspicious cases.

10

MISCELLANEOUS SKIN PROBLEMS

ACRAL LICK DERMATITIS

Acral lick dermatitis, or lick granuloma, is a fairly common condition in which the dog licks at a body part, usually a spot on the legs, until it is raw and sore. The reason why a dog would do this is currently a matter of much debate. Although some researchers suggest that boredom is at the core of the problem, others believe there is a mild nerve disorder (sensory polyneuropathy), and yet others believe it is a neurotic (obsessive-compulsive) disorder. Doberman Pinschers, Great Danes, German Shepherd Dogs, Labrador Retrievers, and Irish Setters are most commonly affected.

Dogs with acral lick dermatitis begin licking at a site, removing the hair, causing inflammation, and finally removing layers of the skin, sometimes down to the bone. The area becomes raw and weeping, and the chronic trauma itself becomes irritating, further stimulating the dog to lick and chew.

Although there is a temptation to make the diagnosis whenever a dog is chewing at its leg for no apparent reason, the diagnosis needs confirmation. Ideally, all suspected cases should have skin scrapings, bacterial and fungal cultures, and biopsies; it is critical not to miss potentially curable disorders that might just resemble acral lick dermatitis.

With true acral lick dermatitis, treatment must be directed at both the skin disorder and any underlying psychological problems. The first step is to address the dog's mental state. Boredom and stress are often cited as factors in the condition, but many researchers liken this abnormal grooming behavior to the abnormal psychiatric behavior in humans with obsessive-compulsive disorder. If the cause cannot be determined, mood-altering drugs such as tranquilizers, female sex hormones (e.g., medroxyprogesterone acetate), antibiotics (e.g., oxacillin), or narcotic antagonists can be used until the skin lesion is cleared up. Pimozide (Orap), a drug used in humans, has also had some limited successes. The narcotic antagonists (drugs used to reverse the effects of narcotics) are receiving a great deal of attention as treatment for this condition. Surprisingly, some success has also been achieved by using narcotics such as hydrocodone. The fact that narcotics as well as the drugs that inhibit their action may both be beneficial in treating this condition only adds to the confusion already surrounding it.

The initial treatment of dogs with acral lick dermatitis usually includes topical treatments and denying them access to the site of the problem. To keep them from reaching their legs, Elizabethan collars or modified buckets may be placed around their heads and secured to their collars. This is not a suitable long-term solution but is frequently necessary for 6–8 weeks to allow the sites time to heal. During this phase, corticosteroids and anti-inflammatory agents, sometimes combined with the penetrating agent DMSO, are applied to the area. This also cannot be continued long-term because of the risk of absorbing the corticosteroids through the skin and into the bloodstream with repeated use. One of the favored combinations to be used during this initial period is a concoction of flunixin meglumine (Banamine), DMSO, and the corticosteroid fluocinolone (Synotic).

Not that long ago, acral lick dermatitis was one of the hardest disorders to treat; everything in the book was prescribed at one time or another, including cobra antivenin injected into the sites, radiation therapy, and orgotein. None of these was completely successful, yet all seemed to work in a small percentage of cases.

Today, most treatment is with the narcotic antagonists, pimozide, and antidepressants such as amitryptiline, clomipramine, and trioxazine for long-term control. Acral lick dermatitis is a hot topic for research, and much progress is likely to be made in the near future.

ALOPECIA

Alopecia refers to an area of skin that, for one reason or another, has less hair than normal. It is a description, not a diagnosis. Like many terms used in veterinary dermatology, alopecia is not specific for any one disorder;

it is a common finding with many different conditions. Consequently, there is not a single treatment for alopecia. Treatment must be directed at the underlying cause.

Some of the inherited forms of alopecia and follicular dysplasias are discussed in the chapter on breed-related skin problems. These actually represent only a small percentage of the cases of hair loss seen in dogs. One of the most important distinctions to be made in dogs with alopecia is whether the hair was removed by licking or scratching, or whether it just fell out. Hair loss is common when dogs have allergies, fleas, keratinization disorders, or any other problem that might be itchy. On the other hand, there are many other conditions that just cause hairs to fall out. This can result from certain parasites (especially demodicosis and *Pelodera dermatitis*), bacterial infections, fungal infections (especially dermatophytosis), immune-mediated disorders (alopecia areata, lupus erythematosus, scleroderma), hormonal skin problems (hypothyroidism, hyperadrenocorticism, growth hormone-responsive dermatosis, sex hormone-related dermatoses), skin cancers (T-cell-like lymphoma, Sertoli-cell tumor), and other problems (sebaceous adenitis, epidermal dysplasia, toxicities, adverse reactions to such drugs as methotrexate and cyclophosphamide, keratinization defects, etc.).

Telogen effluvium (defluxion) refers to hair loss following stressful periods such as severe illness, fever, shock, pregnancy, or surgery. The hairs are forced into a resting stage, and hair loss may be profound before a new wave of hair growth commences 4–8 weeks after the insult.

Pattern baldness is a regional hair loss that may be associated with aging or testosterone levels, or may be breed-related. The ear flaps and topline are usually affected the most, but there is usually no underlying ailment requiring treatment. A patterned alopecia of the trunk has been reported in the Portuguese Water Dog and is currently being studied. Since this appears to be a breed-specific pattern alopecia, biopsies of all affected dogs are recommended so the condition can be better understood.

Periodic alopecia, as its name would indicate, tends to wax and wane over time. It has been seen in a number of breeds, including Poodles, Dachshunds, and Airedales. Airedales may show significant darkening of the skin in alopecic regions. No underlying cause has been determined.

Seasonal alopecia has been reported in Airedales, Boxers, and English Bulldogs. They lose hair on the trunk during the winter, and the skin turns very dark in the affected area. The hair regrows during the spring and summer, but often not entirely to normal length. The cause is unknown, but growth hormone deficiency, sex hormone imbalance, and pineal gland abnormalities have all been suggested.

Traction alopecia is caused when the hair is bound tightly with constrictive devices such as elastics, bows, or barrettes. The constant tugging on the hair shafts can damage the hair follicles and result in hairless patches.

ANAL SAC DISORDERS

The anal sacs, often mistakenly referred to as anal glands, act as reservoirs for the secretions of the anal sac glands. Anal sac secretions are periodically released through two ducts on either side of the rectum. Normal anal sac fluid is brown and slightly granular, and has a distinctly disagreeable odor (an understatement). Presumably the odor and fluid are associated with social recognition and territorial marking among dogs.

Anal sac fluid is normally emptied with each bowel movement, but a number of conditions can impede its release, causing discomfort as the sacs are expanded by their contents, like little balloons. Some factors that make dogs more susceptible to anal sac disease include having a large quantity of thick secretions, an abnormally small duct system, anal irritation, changes in muscle tone or fecal form, and diarrhea or estrus ("heat"). Diarrhea is probably the most common culprit, because it takes a large, solid stool to expand the rectum and compress the sacs so they release their fluid contents. If the sacs are not periodically expressed during defecation, the contents accumulate, become gritty and thick, and encourage bacterial infections. If the ducts become plugged with matter, the sacs are said to be "impacted" and can eventually rupture. If pus accumulates in the sacs they are said to be "abscessed." Through a little-known immunologic mechanism called conditioned hyperirritability, anal sac disorders can even result in itchiness in other parts of the body, including the face, ears, and feet.

It is not uncommon to see dogs with anal sac problems "scoot" on their backsides or chew at the anal area. Anal sacs should be periodically checked and their contents expressed if necessary. The anal sacs, due to their anatomy and location, are prone to a number of disorders, including impaction, infection, abscessation, and cancer.

Impaction, infection, and abscessation of the anal sacs are relatively common in dogs and require little formal diagnostic testing. Bacterial culture and sensitivity tests are sometimes helpful if antibiotics are to be prescribed, but a great many bacteria are normally found in this area, and culture results can be misleading. Microscopic examination of anal sac fluid is quite helpful, since the presence of a large number of white blood cells is a good indicator that the sacs are infected. Biopsies are usually reserved for dogs suspected of having cancers of the anal sacs or the glands that supply them.

Some problems can be treated by expressing the sacs regularly — gently squeezing them so their contents are released into the rectum, where they can't cause problems. Sometimes it is also necessary to "flush" the sacs with antiseptics and antibiotics. With recurrent problems, oral antibiotics may also be necessary.

If anal sac problems persist, it may be necessary to remove them. This is usually limited to cases with severe infection, cancer, or sometimes, perianal fistulae (see chapter on bacterial and fungal skin diseases).

Malignant adenocarcinoma of the anal sac glands is a potentially devastating cancer. It may alter blood levels of calcium and phosphorus and can spread internally. Its early recognition and surgical removal is critical if affected dogs are to be cured. Because of its location, it may go unnoticed; some are found by routine rectal examination during a veterinary visit. Sometimes the only clue is that the dog is having difficulty defecating.

EAR PROBLEMS

Otitis externa, the inflammation of the outer ear canal, is common in dogs. Otitis externa is a description, not a diagnosis. Conditions that encourage it include a long, relatively narrow ear canal, pendulous ears, and hair growth within the ear canal. All of these may contribute to ear problems, but they don't cause them. That is the job of a number of skin diseases, including bacterial, fungal, and yeast infections, parasitic infestations, allergies, autoimmune diseases, nutritional disorders, keratinization disorders, environmental causes, cancer, and foreign objects such as grass awns. The ears are just flaps of skin; therefore, any disease that affects the skin can result in ear problems.

Although the temptation is to blame otitis externa on bacterial or fungal infections, this is only half true. Since the skin is not sterile and bacteria and yeasts are commonly found in the ear canals of normal dogs, these microbes only cause a problem when something else allows them to grow out of control. In the case of the yeast *Malassezia pachydermatitis,* moisture alone can cause it to proliferate and cause inflammation. The most common causes for a microbial population explosion are the presence of ear mites, allergies, hormonal disorders, grass awns, or keratinization abnormalities. If these underlying problems do not get properly diagnosed and treated, don't expect a long-term cure.

It is not usually difficult to diagnose otitis externa. Head shaking is a common feature, as is a painful reaction when the ear is touched. Head shaking may be so pronounced that small blood vessels are damaged and a hematoma forms in the ear flap. Persistent infections or irritations within the ear canal result in a red and very thickened ear canal lining, further narrowing the opening. This makes the problem worse. Secretions in the ear canal may produce a foul smell and recur quickly, even after they have been thoroughly removed by cleaning.

The most sensible approach to otitis externa is for a veterinarian to carefully evaluate the ear canals, all the way to the ear drum. The ear canals should be flushed completely clean and the ear drum carefully inspected. If the eardrum is ruptured, oral antibiotics will be necessary for the middle ear infection (otitis media), and some ear drops will not be safe to use. If the ear drums are intact but the ear canals are swollen and inflamed, combinations of topical antibiotics and corticosteroids may be used for 5–7 days while investigating for underlying causes. By the end of that week, either specific treatment should be commenced or medication should be switched to safer products (e.g., antiseptics rather than antibiotics; hydrocortisone rather than stronger corticosteroids) that are more suitable for long-term use.

Before any medications are instilled into the ear canal, it is critical to determine if the ear drum is intact or ruptured. If the ear drum (tympanum) is ruptured, then any medications put into the external ear canal may pass into the middle ear. This can be dangerous because some agents are known to be ototoxic and can induce hearing loss or disturb balance. This includes antibiotics commonly included in ear drops, creams and ointments, such as neomycin, gentamicin, polymixin B, and chloramphenicol, and antiseptics such as chlorhexidine, iodine, and cetrimide. These products are only meant to be applied into ear canals which have an intact ear drum.

As a final option, ear problems due to chronic lack of ventilation can be surgically corrected. Part of the vertical ear canal is removed, giving the ear canal better exposure. About 50% of dogs that have this surgery improve significantly. Dogs with chronically inflamed and scarred ears or ones in which the horizontal ear canal has been markedly narrowed don't do as well.

For these dogs, another option exists. This is to remove the entire ear canal, an advanced surgical procedure but one that is necessary in some stubborn cases.

Aural hematomas result when blood vessels burst in the ear flaps and the blood collects between the skin and cartilage. There has been a long-standing discussion as to why this affects some dogs and not others, but no clear-cut reasons have been proposed. It is generally accepted that most dogs have an ear problem first, then shake their heads, which damages the blood vessels in the ear flaps. Another theory is that dogs prone to developing aural hematomas have an immune-mediated disorder; this has been suggested because some animals can be successfully treated with corticosteroids. The most common form of therapy is surgical drainage of the collected blood and "tacking down" the skin so that no space is left for more blood to pool.

Pinnal hair loss, a baldness of the ear flaps, may be seen with a number of conditions, including pinnal alopecia (seen most commonly in Dachshunds, Chihuahuas, and Whippets), periodic alopecia (seen in Poodles), and congenito-hereditary disorders. Hormonal disorders (hypothyroidism, sex hormone imbalances), dermatophytosis, demodicosis, and alopecia areata may or may not be associated with inflammation in the outer ear. The pinnae may also be involved in a number of generalized skin diseases, including allergic inhalant dermatitis, food allergy, ear-margin dermatosis, cutaneous vasculitis, pemphigus erythematosus and foliaceus, systemic and discoid lupus erythematosus, dermatomyositis, lichenoid dermatoses, and keratinization disorders.

ENVIRONMENTAL CAUSES
OF SKIN DISEASE

Solar dermatitis is implicated in many different skin diseases and is covered in more detail in its own section below. Sun damage to skin has been associated with nasal solar dermatitis, actinic keratosis, elastosis, and several skin cancers, including squamous-cell carcinoma and hemangiosarcoma. Solar radiation also worsens (but doesn't cause) symptoms associated with lupus erythematosus and a variety of other depigmenting diseases.

Irritant contact dermatitis and its similarity to allergic contact dermatitis is discussed in the chapter on allergies. Primary irritants to dog skin include acids, alkalis, soaps, detergents, fertilizers, herbicides, insecticides, and even flea collars. The problem is caused not by an allergic reaction but rather by the caustic effect of an ingredient on the skin. The areas most affected are those with the sparsest haircoat, including the belly, ears, scrotum, and feet. These areas become red and itchy and are often bitten and scratched. Sometimes the diagnosis can be deduced from the history alone (e.g., happened right after a bath with a new shampoo), but often biopsies and patch testing are required. Treatment involves thoroughly cleansing the skin and coat with a gentle hypoallergenic shampoo and avoiding the contact irritant in the future. A short corse of corticosteroids is sometimes necessary to help control the inflammation in the skin.

Burns are as serious on dog skin as they are on human skin. Burns are also frequently complicated by microbial infections and sepsis, which can be life-threatening. The most common causes of burns in dogs are hot water, heating pads, hair dryers, and fires. Since the skin of dogs is covered by fur, burns are not always apparent as soon as they occur. It may be days before the dog is taken to a veterinarian. By this time the burned skin has become thick and dry and infection is evident beneath the dead skin. Eventually the skin sloughs in this area and leaves an open wound. If more than 25% of the body surface is involved, internal complications (e.g., shock, sepsis, kidney failure, respiratory distress, anemia, etc.) are to be expected. The treatment for burns in dogs includes supportive care (fluid therapy, keeping the dog warm, highly digestible diet), removing debris and dead skin, and thorough cleansing with an approved antiseptic. Then the burn should be cleaned daily, and suitable antibiotics (e.g., silver sulfadiazine) should be applied. Burns heal slowly, and if the full thickness of the skin was damaged, there will be scarring and permanent hair loss.

Frostbite is common in dogs that have been left outdoors during freezing weather. It principally affects the ears, tail, toes, and scrotum, and the damage caused to the skin often resembles that of a burn. Once dogs are rescued, warm water should be used to rapidly thaw the frozen tissues; gentleness is very important to minimize pain and tissue damage. For animals with severe damage, surgery may be necessary to remove dead tissue.

Poisonings (toxicoses) are occasionally responsible for causing skin problems. Although the rodent poison thallium is no longer available in North America, thallium poisonings still occasionally happen here. Arsenic poisoning can also create skin problems; it is included in many herbicides, rodent poisons, pesticides, and some medications. Poisoning can cause a number of different dermatologic manifestations, including hair loss, inflamed skin, bruising, and sometimes, bleeding.

FOOTPAD DISEASES

Diseased footpads are often referred to as hyperkeratotic footpads, since the pads tend to become thickened, cracked, and scaly when diseased. Footpad diseases have various causes. In the past, many cases were undoubtedly due to distemper (hard pad disease). However, since the advent of modern vaccination programs, distemper is now rare.

Today, many different conditions are known to cause footpad disorders, including parasitism (hookworms, *Pelodera*), bacterial infections, fungal infections (dermatophytes, yeasts, intermediate and deep fungi), contact allergy, autoimmune diseases (lupus erythematosus, pemphigus foliaceus), nutritional skin diseases (zinc-responsive dermatosis, generic dog food disease), congenito-hereditary diseases (lethal acrodermatitis, tyrosinemia), neoplasms (squamous-cell carcinoma), foreign body penetration, contact irritation, acral mutilation syndrome, and nasodigital hyperkeratosis.

Acral mutilation syndrome is a bizarre inherited condition most commonly seen in Pointer pups. Possibly because of abnormal nerve supply to their feet, they chew their legs to the point of mutilation. This is covered in more detail in the chapter on breed-related skin problems.

Lethal acrodermatitis, also covered in more detail in the chapter on breed-related skin problems, is a syndrome in Bull Terriers characterized by growth retardation, infection of the feet, chronic pyoderma and nailbed disease, diarrhea, pneumonia, abnormal behavior, and death by 16 months of age. Recently, some mildly affected cases have been maintained on ketoconazole, a drug used to treat deep fungal infections.

Familial vasculopathy is the tentative name given to a recently described footpad disease syndrome seen in German Shepherd Dogs. The disease itself may be inherited, or it may be that an inherited immune problem causes these dogs to react adversely when vaccinated. At this point, there are more questions than answers. At very young ages (less than 6 months), these dogs develop swollen feet and often crusts and scales on their noses, lips, and ear margins. Pigment may also be lost from the footpads and nose. Dogs may also be lethargic, lame, and occasionally have a fever. To date, diagnosis has relied on biopsies and immunologic testing. Treatment with corticosteroids usually allows the dogs to walk more easily, and it appears that many improve spontaneously at 5–6 months of age. There is some concern that these recovered dogs may be prone to an internal disease, amyloidosis, when they are 2 or 3 years old.

Tyrosinemia, a rare metabolic disese, has also been reported in a German Shepherd Dog. The footpads and nose became thick and ulcerated, and there was a related eye disease. The diagnosis is based on skin biopsies and on finding high levels of tyrosine in the blood and urine. Treatment is supportive and includes a low-phenylalanine, low-tyrosine diet.

Nasodigital hyperkeratosis is a strange ailment in which excessive layers of the shingle-like keratin accumulate on the nose and/or footpads. The cause is unknown. The condition is diagnosed by excluding the other causes that have already been discussed. Treatment is attempted by shaving away the excess dead tissue and applying hydrating ointments to increase shedding of the accumulated material.

INTERNAL DISEASES THAT MAY AFFECT THE SKIN

Not all skin problems originate in the skin. A number of them reflect an internal problem.

Nodular dermatofibrosis, described in the chapter on skin tumors, is a harmless skin eruption that occurs in German Shepherd Dogs in association with a cancerous problem of the kidneys or uterus.

Superficial necrolytic dermatitis, also known as diabetic dermatopathy, hepatic dermatopathy, hepatocutaneous syndrome, glucagonoma syndrome, and necrolytic migratory erythema, was discussed in the chapter on keratinization disorders. It may be caused by diabetes mellitus, liver/gall bladder disease, kidney disease, pancreatic disease, cancer, defects of bile acid and uric acid metabolism, and a variety of other disorders. Affected dogs usually have laboratory evidence of liver disease, high levels of glucagon (a hormone with effects opposite to insulin), glucose intolerance, and low blood levels of albumin, an important protein in the blood. There are currently no general treatments available (except surgery in the case of tumors of the pancreas), but amino acid therapies are being investigated. Treatment must always be directed at the underlying causative problem.

Sepsis, a severe internal bacterial infection, can occasionally result in bruises, ulcers, and pimples on the skin surface as bacteria and their toxins exert their effects. Diagnosis is made by skin biopsy and by microbial culture of the skin and blood. Treatment is directed at the life-threatening internal infection.

Atypical microbial infections such as plague, tuberculosis, nocardiosis, and the systemic fungal infections may cause skin problems (lumps and sores), but their primary target is usually internal organs, principally the lungs. From here they may spread outward to many organs, including the skin. Diagnosis is made by x-rays, blood tests, biopsy/cytology, and appropriate cultures. Treatment is directed at the systemic infection, not just the skin.

Parasitic infections such as tick-borne diseases (babesiosis, Rocky Mountain spotted fever, ehrlichiosis, Lyme disease), heartworm, leishmaniasis, and toxoplasmosis are primarily systemic (internal) diseases that occasionally may cause skin problems (bumps, bruises, lumps). Diagnosis and treatment is directed at the internal parasite.

Viral infections can also result in skin problems. Other than the papilloma (wart) virus, which is limited to surface epithelium, most viruses begin by causing internal disease, then occasionally later affecting the skin. The distemper virus can cause thickening and scaling of the footpads and nose (hard pad disease). The paravaccinia virus, which principally affects sheep and goats, can also infect dogs that eat infected carcasses.

NAIL AND NAILBED DISEASES

Diseases of the nails and nailbeds are uncommon in dogs, but when they do occur, they are often difficult to diagnose and treat. The nails (more correctly termed claws) and nailbeds (ungual folds) may be affected by bacterial infections (paronychia), fungal infections (onychomycosis), yeast infections (*Candida* paronychia), autoimmune disorders (lupus erythematosus), inherited defects, nutritional imbalances, cardiopulmonary disease, and parasites (demodicosis). Many things can happen to the claws, and each problem is called by a different name.

Among claw diseases, bacterial paronychia is not uncommon, but the underlying cause may be difficult to uncover. It is very rare indeed for dogs to have infected claws without some other predisposing cause. Immune system disorders that can make the claws prone to infection include systemic lupus erythematosus, vasculitis, pemphigus vulgaris, bullous pemphigoid, lupoid dermatosis, erythema multiforme, and drug eruption.

Onychomycosis, fungal infection of the claws, may occur with dermatophytosis, sporotrichosis, blastomycosis, and yeasts. The diagnosis is based on cultures, cytologic examination, and biopsies. The condition is usually treated with ketoconazole (Nystatin for *Candida* yeasts), which must be used for many months to be completely successful. Antiseptic flushes are also recommended.

The term onychorrhexis describes brittle nails, most commonly caused by chronic low-grade infection. Other causes can be genetic, nutritional, or senile changes. It is most commonly noticed in young German Shepherd Dogs, Rhodesian Ridgebacks, Dachshunds, and Cocker Spaniels, as well as in older dogs of many breeds. If the underlying problem can be identified, treatment should be aimed at that, and the nails should be filed rather than trimmed.

Onychomadesis is sloughing of the claw. Causes include a multitude of immune-mediated disorders (lupus erythematosus, pemphigus, pemphigoid), loss of blood supply to the claw, trauma, and infection. Arriving at a diagnosis is not always a simple matter. In addition to a thorough physical examination, blood counts, biochemical profiles, cultures, urinalysis, and antinuclear antibody tests should be done. Heart function may also need to be checked.

Treatment can also be complicated. The bacteria can often be managed by appropriate antibiotic therapy and antiseptic flushes. Unfortunately, if an underlying cause cannot be identified, antibiotics may need to be used long-term. An alternative is the surgical removal of the nails. Nutritional supplementation with zinc, methionine, or gelatin (Knox gelatin in food at 1 packet/15 lb. body weight daily) may help some affected dogs. Combinations of tetracycline and niacinamide have been used to treat some of the immune-mediated causes of onychomadesis.

NASAL DERMATITIS

Nasal dermatitis describes a number of very different conditions that affect the skin of the nose. It was formerly referred to as "Collie nose," which is inappropriate, since any breed may be affected. It was also thought that the cause of the problem was excessive sun exposure, but that has proven to be rarely the case. In fact, it is now known that many different diseases can result in nasal dermatitis; therefore, correct treatment depends on diagnosis of the underlying cause.

Conditions that can cause nasal dermatitis include external parasites (especially demodectic mange), bacterial infections (nasal pyoderma, dermatophilosis), fungal infections (dermatophytosis, intermediate and deep mycoses), allergies (inhalant, food, contact), autoimmune skin diseases (pemphigus foliaceus, pemphigus erythematosus, bullous pemphigoid, systemic and discoid lupus erythematosus, Vogt-Koyanagi-Harada-like syndrome), nutritional skin diseases (vitamin A-responsive dermatosis, zinc-responsive dermatosis, generic dog food disease), neoplasms (cutaneous T-cell lymphoma, squamous-cell carcinoma), hereditary diseases (dermatomyositis, epidermolysis bullosa simplex, tyrosinemia), trauma, drug eruption, and photodermatitis (a reaction to sun exposure).

For a dog with nasal dermatitis, a step-by-step approach should be taken so that a proper diagnosis can be made and suitable treatment instituted. This might include skin scrapings (looking for parasites), bacterial and fungal cultures, and ideally, biopsies. Other tests may be performed as warranted. Treatment must be directed at the specific cause.

PODODERMATITIS

Pododermatitis is a descriptive term denoting inflammation of the feet and the spaces between the toes. One or more feet may be involved. As is often the case, inflammation is caused by a variety of different disorders. Dogs that frequently get pododermatitis should be evaluated for possible allergy (inhalant, food), hypothyroidism, dermatophytosis, immune-mediated diseases, and immunoincompetence.

Interdigital pyoderma is covered in the chapter on bacterial and fungal skin problems, and sterile pyogranuloma is covered in the chapter on immune-mediated skin disorders. These two conditions account for the vast majority of cases of pododermatitis. In most cases, there is redness between the toes, and eventually lumps develop in these sites and may bleed or discharge pus. Despite the fact that most owners think the problem is caused by "cysts," this is only rarely the case. Most of the time these "cysts" turn out to be nodules of infection and inflammation. The breeds most commonly affected with pododermatitis include English Bulldogs, Great Danes, Boxers, Doberman Pinschers, Rottweilers, Chinese Shar-peis, Dachshunds, and Labrador Retrievers.

The proper diagnosis of pododermatitis is difficult, because diagnostic tests aren't always helpful. Virtually all cases, regardless of actual cause, eventually are overrun by bacteria. This confuses the picture, because the bacteria can camouflage the real problem. Unfortunately, what frequently happens is that antibiotics are prescribed for one to two months and the feet often look much improved. Shortly after the antibiotics are discontinued, however, the problem comes back. This is a good indication that the bacteria were complicating, not causing the problem, and the search for a cure must continue.

True pyodermas respond to appropriate doses and intervals of antibiotics. Sterile pyogranuloma often responds very well to moderate doses of corticosteroids. Chronic deep interdigital pyoderma and immunodeficiencies do not usually have a happy ending. Sometimes, even surgery is needed to remove some of the more inflamed tissue. In especially stubborn cases, all the affected tissues can be removed, effectively fusing the dog's toes. This is referred to as a fusion podoplasty.

PRURITUS

Pruritus (itchiness) is probably the number one reason for dog owners to seek veterinary attention. Dogs that scratch can not only do considerable damage to their skin but are often disruptive to the household. After being kept awake for a few nights by a scratching dog, owners want instant relief and may not be agreeable to postponing treatment until a diagnosis is made.

There is little doubt that most itchy dogs have allergies and/or fleas, but clearly, these aren't the only reasons for itchiness. Bacterial and fungal infections, keratinization disorders, immune-mediated diseases, and even cancers can be itchy if given half a chance.

All itchy dogs should be searched for fleas, but if none are found, that still doesn't let fleas off the hook. In flea-allergic dogs, it only takes the bite of one flea every 5–7 days to cause a perpetual problem. Since for every flea you see on a dog there are likely 100–300 in the immediate environment, never seeing a flea on the dog does not mean they are not causing the problem. The theory can be tested by allergy-testing for flea bite hypersensitivity or by doing an insecticide trial. See the chapter on parasites for more information about fleas and flea control.

The most common diagnostic test done on itchy dogs is a skin scraping. A dulled scalpel blade is lubricated with mineral oil, then the surface layers of the skin are scraped with it and the debris is collected and evaluated by microscope. This test is not foolproof, but is one of the best tests for finding a variety of mites that may be responsible for the itchiness. Unfortunately, in some forms of mange (the skin problems caused by mites), the mites are exceptionally difficult to find and are only uncovered perhaps a third of the time. A modified skin scraping procedure can also be done to search for yeasts (especially *Malassezia pachydermatis*), another cause of intense itchiness in dogs.

Allergies are exceptionally common in dogs, especially purebreds, and other than fleas, are the most likely cause of itchiness in dogs. Allergic inhalant dermatitis (atopy) is the canine version of hay fever, and the itchiness is an allergic reaction to a variety of pollens, molds, house dust, and danders. Food allergy and food intolerance are less common than inhalant allergies but must be considered in the itchy pet, especially if the symptoms are year-round. Allergies are covered in much more detail in the chapter on allergic skin disorders.

Bacterial infections of the skin are common and can also be itchy; so can fungal infections. Sometimes the infection is itchy all by itself and sometimes it is itchy as a result of an allergic reaction to the microbe.

Keratinization disorders, conditions that cause the skin to be dry or greasy, are frequently itchy because the skin beocmes thickened and because they encourage the growth of microbes on the skin surface.

In looking at the reasons for dogs to be itchy, it becomes obvious that almost anything can make a dog want to scratch. It is important to identify the correct cause of the itchiness so that the most appropriate form of therapy can be used. If a diagnosis is not reached, corticosteroids are frequently a part of the treatment regimen. Because of their potential side effects, they should be used cautiously. Happily, an underlying cause for most cases of pruritis can be found and appropriately managed.

For most itchy dogs, at least some relief can be gained by cool-water baths using gentle ingredients like oatmeal, sulfur, salicylic acid, or selenium sulfide. These baths need to be given frequently to be effective, sometimes daily if the symptoms are severe. This is not necessarily convenient for long-term management but does help in the short term while the pieces of the puzzle are being assembled. A variety of safe sprays are also available to help temporarily relieve itching; most include pH-balanced hamamelis (witch hazel) and/or hydrocortisone. Stronger preparations should only be used for periods of less than ten days, and only under veterinary direction.

SOLAR DERMATITIS

Solar dermatitis, or photodermatitis, is seen on the sparsely haired regions of dogs with light-colored skin. Areas that are well covered by fur are protected from solar damage, so this condition is seen mainly on the top of the nose and on the belly. Although it may occur anywhere geographically, this is more a problem in dogs living in parts of the country that are particularly sunny.

There appears to be significant differences between the pattern of damage on the nose and on the belly. To develop solar dermatitis on the top of the nose, there must be light-colored skin; many affected dogs are born with less than adequate pigment in this region. This part of the nose may therefore initially appear pink or white. With time and repeated exposure to ultraviolet light, the nose develops a rash, and the skin can become severely damaged. A small percentage of dogs can even develop cancers in these areas. See the discussion of nasal dermatitis above in this chapter for information on the more common causes of nasal dermatitis.

Because nasal solar dermatitis resembles so many of the other disorders that affect this area, biopsies should be taken. Treatment of true nasal solar dermatitis involves avoiding exposure to sunlight during peak daylight hours or protecting the area. Sunscreens are helpful, but many dogs lick them off before they can be effective or resist having them applied. Tattooing the area with black ink can also help absorb ultraviolet light.

Solar dermatitis in other areas, principally the belly, is seen in dogs with lightly pigmented skin that like to "sunbathe" or are exposed to sunlight reflected off snow cover. Since affected skin must not only be lightly pigmented but also not covered with protective fur, this form of solar dermatitis is most commonly seen in Bull Terriers, Beagles, and Dalmatians. At first, the skin changes just look like sunburn, and, if you look closely, only white skin is affected. Any black skin in the area remains relatively normal. In time, usually several years, affected dogs may develop "solar elastosis," actinic keratoses, and even skin cancers. Treatment includes keeping these dogs away from direct sun exposure and protecting them with sunscreens. It has also been reported that beta-carotene and anti-inflammatory doses of prednisone can be helpful in reducing inflammation. Any skin cancers should be surgically removed and evaluated by a pathologist.

GLOSSARY

Every attempt has been made to use everyday language in this book along with dermatologic terms. To provide a convenient dictionary of terms, the following glossary includes most of the words commonly used in the science of veterinary dermatology.

ABSCESS. A cavity filled with pus.

ACANTHOSIS. Thickening of the epidermis. Also referred to as epidermal hyperplasia.

ACRAL. The outermost parts of the body, especially the legs.

ALBINISM. An inherited absence of pigment in the skin, hair, and eyes.

ALLERGEN. A substance capable of causing an allergy.

ALLERGY. A heightened sensitivity to substances.

ALOPECIA. Hair loss.

ANEMIA. A condition in which red blood cells are in lower numbers than normal.

ANTHROPOPHILIC. Organisms adapted to live on people. Most commonly used to describe ringworm fungi that prefer people to animals.

ANTIBODY. A substance produced by lymphocytes (actually plasma cells) that protects the body; part of the immune system.

ANTIBIOTIC. A substance that inhibits the growth of microorganisms.

ANTIGEN. A substance capable of causing the production of antibody.

ANTINUCLEAR ANTIBODY. A group of substances that react against cellular components; a common screening test for lupus erythematosus but positive in other conditions as well.

ANTISEPTIC. A substance that inhibits or destroys microorganisms, usually on living tissue.

APOCRINE. The most common form of "sweat gland" in the dog.

143

ATOPY. Another name for inhalant allergies in dogs. Not identical to the condition in people.

AUROTRICHIA. A condition in which the hairs turn golden in color.

AUTOANTIBODY. An antibody directed against part of the body. For instance, thyroid autoantibody targets thyroid glandular elements.

AUTOGENOUS. Originating from the animal's own body, such as an autogenous vaccine made up of bacteria harvested directly from the animal to be treated. This is sometimes done for staphylococcal infections and for viral "warts."

AUTOIMMUNE. A process whereby the body directs antibodies against part of itself.

BASAL CELLS. The bottom row of cells in the epidermis. They produce keratinocytes that eventually die and form the surface scale.

BENIGN. Harmless.

BIOPSY. Removing tissue from living patients for diagnostic evaluation.

BULLA. A large blister.

CELLULITIS. Inflammation of the connective tissue; a diffuse infection compared to the abscess that comes to a "head."

CERUMEN. A wax-like secretion found in the ear canal.

CHEMOTHERAPY. Treatment of disease by chemical substances or drugs.

CHRYSTOTHERAPY. Treatment of disease with gold compounds.

COLLAGEN. The fibrous connective tissue of the dermis; the supportive network of the skin.

COMPLEMENT. A group of compounds that act in sequence to bring about the destruction of foreign substances; part of the immune response.

CONGENITAL. A feature present at birth that may or may not be hereditary.

CORTICOSTEROID. Family of steroid hormones that are related to cortisone.

CRUST. A scab.

CRYOSURGERY. Surgery utilizing very cold temperatures such as that produced by liquid nitrogen or carbon dioxide.

CUTIS. Another name for skin.

CYTOLOGY. The diagnostic evaluation of individual cells, rather than tissue.

CYTOPLASM. The part of a cell outside of the nucleus.

DEPIGMENTATION. Loss of color (pigment) from the skin.

DERMAL-EPIDERMAL JUNCTION. The area between the dermis and epidermis.

DERMAL PAPILLA. A structure formed by the dermis to provide nutrition and a blood supply to a developing hair follicle.

DERMATOLOGY. The study of skin disorders.

DERMATOPHYTE. A ringworm-causing fungus.

DERMATOPHYTOSIS. Superficial fungal infection; ringworm.

DERMIS. That fibrous part of the skin located between the epidermis and the subcutaneous fat.

ECCRINE. An uncommon type of sweat gland in the dog, located only on the nose and footpads.

ECZEMA. A family of inflammatory rashes with various other clinical features.

ELECTROSURGERY. Cutting and cautery provided by an electric current.

ELISA. Enzyme-linked immunosorbent assay. A technique used in diagnostic testing.

EMOLLIENT. An agent that softens the skin or soothes irritation.

ENDOCRINOLOGY. The study of hormones.

EOSINOPHIL. A type of white blood cell often conspicuous in parasitic and allergic conditions.

EPIDERMAL COLLARETTE. A peeling edge of scale surrounding what once was a fluid-filled structure, such as a pimple or blister.

EPIDERMIS. The uppermost layer of the skin formed by rows of keratinocytes.

EROSION. A shallow defect in the skin that does not penetrate as far as the dermis.

ERYTHEMA. Redness.

ERYTHRODERMA. An inflammatory reaction in the skin often accompanied by redness and scaling.

ETIOLOGY. Cause.

EXFOLIATE. To shed skin cells or surface scale.

EXUDATION. The oozing of material through the skin, e.g., pus, serum.

FAMILIAL. A trait that runs in families.

FISTULA. An abnormal tract leading from a site of infection to the surface of the skin.

FOLLICULITIS. Infection of hair follicles.

FOMITES. Substances such as bedding, grooming instruments, etc., capable of absorbing and transmitting infections. Example: ringworm can be spread between animals on fomites.

FURUNCULOSIS. Marked folliculitis resulting in rupture of the hair follicle.

GEOPHILIC. Organisms that have become adapted specifically to live in the environment. Most commonly used to describe ringworm fungi that prefer the soil to animals or people.

GRANULOMA. A lump in the skin caused by the body "walling off" substances with special white blood cells called histiocytes (macrophages).

GROUND SUBSTANCE. The gel-like matrix of the dermis.

GUARD HAIRS. The long, primary hairs of animals.

HEMATOMA. A pocket of blood formed in tissue.

HERITABLE. A trait that can be inherited; transmitted by genetic material.

HISTOPATHOLOGY. The microscopic examination of abnormal tissue.

HOT SPOT. A localized, superficial bacterial infection.

HYPERPIGMENTATION. Increased pigmentation in the skin.

HYPERSENSITIVITY. Increased sensitivity to substances.

HYPODERMIS. Same as subcutis, the fat layer underlying the dermis.

HYPOSENSITIZATION. A form of immunotherapy whereby sensitivity to substances is alleviated by a series of injections designed to moderate the immune response. Example: allergy shots.

HYPOTRICHOSIS. Less hair than normal.

IATROGENIC. Disorder caused by medical intervention. Example: iatrogenic Cushing's disease is caused when too much cortisone is administerred to a patient.

IDIOPATHIC. Of unknown cause.

IMMUNOFLUORESCENCE. A diagnostic procedure in which autoantibodies are identified by substances that glow and act as markers.

IMMUNOGLOBULIN. A family of antibodies.

IMMUNOPATHOLOGY. The study of immune-mediated diseases using substances that identify autoantibodies in tissues, including immunofluorescence and immuno-peroxidase studies.

IMMUNOPEROXIDASE. A diagnostic procedure whereby autoantibodies are identified by peroxidase, a form of stain.

IMMUNOTHERAPY. Treatment directed at the production of protective immunity. Most common example is allergy shots but also used in the treatment of some bacterial infections, viral infections, fungal infections, and cancers.

IMPETIGO. A superficial bacterial infection of dogs which is significantly different than the human condition with the same name.

INFECTION. A condition in which microorganisms flourish on or within the body.

INFESTATION. A condition in which parasites are dwelling on the surface of the skin.

INFLAMMATION. Redness and swelling in tissue.

INTERLEUKINS. Substances produced by cells that promote or suppress inflammation.

INTRADERMAL. Injection into the dermis

KERATIN. The proteins that form the shingle-like stratum corneum covering the epidermis.

KERATINIZATION. The process in which the epidermal cells (keratinocytes) evolve from living cells to the dead cells that form the stratum corneum, the surface scale.

KERATINOCYTE. An epidermal cell that eventually dies to contribute to the stratum corneum, the scale on the surface of the skin.

KERATOCONJUNCTIVITIS SICCA. A deficiency of tears; dry eye.

LANGERHANS' CELL. A cell present in the epidermis that is important in immune regulation.

LESION. Any deviation from normal tissue.

LEUKOTRIENE. A substance produced by cells that causes or regulates some forms of inflammation.

LICHENIFICATION. A thickening and hardening of the skin with exaggerated folding. It is often referred to as resembling the skin of an elephant.

LYMPHOCYTE. A type of white blood cell. B-lymphocytes go on to become plasma cells that produce antibodies. T-lymphocytes patrol the body, guarding against invasion.

LYMPHOKINE. A substance produced by lymphocytes; important in the immune response.

MACROPHAGE. A tissue cell important in immune regulation. In a different form (histiocyte) this cell is important in the formation of granulomas.

MACULE. A small (less than 1 cm) flat, colored spot on the skin.

MALIGNANT. A process that tends to get worse. Often used to describe cancers that are likely to cause the most problems.

MANGE. A disease caused by mites.

METASTASIS. The spreading of a disease from one part of the body to another. Usually used to describe the spread of cancer.

MONOCYTE. A white blood cell that is a member of the mononuclear-phagocyte family, related to the tissue macrophage and the histiocyte.

MONOGENIC. Traits controlled by one set of genes.

MONOKINE. A substance produced by members of the mononuclear-phagocyte system; important in the immune response.

MYCOSIS. A disease caused by fungi.

MYIASIS. The invasion of tissues by maggots.

NECROSIS. The death of cells or tissues in a living animal.

NEOPLASIA. A "new growth" or tumor, either benign or malignant.

NEOPLASM. Literally, a "new growth"; usually synonymous with tumor.

NEUTROPHIL. A white blood cell often prominent in bacterial infections.

NODULE. A solid mass extending deeply into the dermis.

NUCLEUS. The rounded or oval mass of genetic material (DNA) located in a cell; separate from the surrounding cytoplasm.

ONCOLOGY. The study of cancers and their treatment.

ONYCHOMADESIS. Sloughing of the nails (claws).

ONYCHOMYCOSIS. A nail (claw) disease caused by fungi.

ONYCHORRHEXIS. Brittle nails (claws).

OTOSCOPE. An instrument designed for examination of the ear canals.

PANNICULITIS. An inflammatory reaction in the subcutaneous fat.

PANNICULUS. Another name for subcutis, the fat layer underneath the dermis.

PAPULE. A small (less than 1 cm) solid elevation of the skin. A bump.

PARASITE. A life-form that draws its nourishment from living in or on another life-form.

PATCH. A large (greater than 1 cm) macule or colored area on the skin.

PATHOGENESIS. The origin or development of a disease.

PHOTODERMATITIS. An inflammatory reaction in the skin due to exposure to sunlight.

PLAQUE. A large (greater than 1 cm) papule.

PLASMA. The fluid portion of the blood.

PODODERMATITIS. Inflammation of the feet.

POLIOSIS. Graying of the hair.

POLYDIPSIA. Increased thirst.

POLYGENIC. Traits controlled by many sets of genes.

POLYPHAGIA. Increased hunger.

POLYURIA. Increased urination.

PROGNOSIS. A forecase of the probable outcome of a disease.

PRURITUS. Itchiness.

PUSTULE. A small, solid elevation of the skin filled with pus; a pimple.

PYODERMA. A bacterial infection of the skin in which pus may be produced.

PYOTRAUMATIC DERMATITIS. A superficial bacterial infection; hot spots.

RAST. Radioallergosorbent testing; a technology used in diagnostic testing.

RESISTANCE. In bacteriology, a state whereby microorganisms are not sufficiently affected by an antibiotic to inhibit their growth.

RINGWORM. Poor term for a superficial fungal infection of the skin.

SCALE. An accumulation of loose fragments of stratum corneum on the skin surface.

SCAR. A fibrous tissue that replaces damaged dermis.

SCLEROSIS. Hardening or thickening.

SEBORRHEA. A catch-all term to describe dogs with dry, greasy, or smelly skin. A keratinization disorder.

SEBUM. The waxy, oily product of the sebaceous glands, which is excreted into the hair follicles and ends up on the skin surface.

SENSITIVITY. In bacteriology, a state in which the growth of microorganisms is inhibited by an antibiotic.

SERUM. The fluid portion of the blood after the clot of blood cells has been removed.

STEROID. A large family of chemicals, including hormones, some vitamins, and drugs.

STRATUM. A layer.

STRATUM CORNEUM. The shingle-like covering of the epidermis.

SUBCUTIS. The layer of fat underlying the dermis.

TARDIVE. An inherited trait that is not manifested at birth but that appears at some later time.

THERMOREGULATION. The ability to regulate temperature.

TITER (OR TITRE). Serum levels of antibodies against specific entities, which may be viral, bacterial, fungal, or immunologic in origin.

TOPICAL. Applied to the surface of the skin.

TOXIN. A poisonous substance.

TUMEFACTION. A swelling.

TUMOR. A swelling, but usually regarding a form of neoplasia.

ULCER. A local defect that penetrates into the dermis.

URTICARIA. Hives.

VASCULITIS. Inflammatory reaction of the blood vessels.

VELLUS HAIRS. The soft downy undercoat of animals.

VESICLE. A blister.

VIBRISSAE. Sensory hairs; whiskers.

VITILIGO. Localized loss of pigment on the skin.

WHEAL. A hive.

XEROSIS. Dryness.

XEROSTOMIA. Dryness of the mouth.

ZOONOSIS. A disease that may be transmitted from animals to humans.

ZOOPHILIC. Pertaining to organisms that have become adapted specifically to animals.

APPENDIX A

LISTING OF COMMON CONDITIONS

This list is included to assist the reader in locating the possible condition causing a skin problem in a particular area. This list is far from conclusive. There are over 500 conditions that could cause itching, for example. However, you may find this list helpful as a starting point when researching a particular problem.

Conditions Most Often Involving the Face

Parasites: demodicosis, trombiculiasis, fly bites, cuterebriasis, Dirofilaria dermatitis

Bacteria: skin-fold pyoderma, pyotraumatic dermatitis, acne, nasal pyoderma, atypical mycobacteriosis

Fungi: hyalohyphomycosis, cryptococcosis

Immune: Allergic inhalant dermatitis, food hypersensitivity, contact dermatitis, lupus erythematosus, pemphigus foliaceus/erythematosus, Vogt-Koyanagi-Harada-like syndrome

Neoplasia: squamous-cell carcinoma, hemangiosarcoma, malignant histiocytosis, fibrous histiocytoma, actinic keratosis, melanoma, papilloma, transmissible venereal tumor

Other: zinc-responsive dermatosis, dermatomyositis, epidermolysis bullosa simplex, spiculosis, viral papillomatosis, juvenile cellulitis, metabolic dermatosis

149

Conditions Most Often Affecting the Nose

Parasites: demodicosis, cuterebriasis, cutaneous dirofilariasis
Bacteria: nasal pyoderma, dermatophilosis, actinomycotic mycetoma
Fungi: dermatophytosis, hyalohyphomycosis, rhinosporidiosis, blastomycosis, coccidioidomycosis, cryptococcosis, histoplasmosis
Immune: allergic inhalant dermatitis, food allergy, contact sensitivity, lupus erythematosus, pemphigus foliaceus/erythematosus, bullous pemphigoid, Vogt-Koyanagi-Harada-like syndrome, drug eruption
Neoplasia: malignant histiocytosis, transmissible venereal tumor, cutaneous T-cell lymphoma, squamous-cell carcinoma
Other: vitamin A-responsive dermatosis, zinc-responsive dermatosis, generic dog food disease, dermatomyositis, epidermolysis bullosa simplex, tyrosinemia, lupoid dermatosis, trauma, photodermatitis, nasodigital hyperkeratosis

Conditions Most Often Involving the Eyelids

Parasites: demodicosis, sarcoptic mange
Bacteria: juvenile pyoderma, bacterial blepharitis
Fungi: dermatophytosis, intermediate mycoses, blastomycosis
Immune: pemphigus, pemphigoid, lupus erythematosus, dermatomyositis, Vogt-Koyanagi-Harada-like syndrome, allergic inhalant dermatitis, food hypersensitivity, parasite hypersensitivity, drug eruption
Endocrine: hypothyroidism, hyperadrenocorticism
Nutritional: vitamin A-responsive dermatosis, zinc-responsive dermatosis, generic dog food disease
Neoplasia: cutaneous lymphoma, T-cell-like lymphoma, acrocordon, squamous-cell carcinoma, adenocarcinoma
Miscellaneous: irritation, seborrheic dermatitis, thallium toxicosis

Conditions Most Often Involving the Head

Parasites: flea infestation, cuterebriasis
Bacteria: pyotraumatic dermatitis, atypical mycobacteriosis
Fungi: dermatophytosis, intermediate mycoses
Immune: pemphigus foliaceus/erythematosus, lupus erythematosus
Neoplasia: basal-cell tumor, histiocytoma, actinic keratosis, collagenous nevi, nodular dermatofibrosis, papilloma, sebaceous-gland hyperplasia, apocrine cyst
Other: zinc-responsive dermatosis, dermatomyositis, epidermolysis, bullosa simplex, juvenile cellulitis, sebaceous adenitis, lupoid dermatosis, subcorneal pustular dermatosis

Conditions Most Often Involving the Ears

Parasites: tick infestation, lice infestation, demodicosis, sarcoptic mange, otodectic mange (ear mites), fly bites

Immune: allergic inhalant dermatitis, pemphigus foliaceus/erythematosus, lupus erythematosus, cutaneous vasculitis, cold agglutinin disease
Other: dermatomyositis, histiocytoma, psoriasiform-lichenoid dermatitis, idiopathic lichenoid dermatitis, hyperestrogenism, pinnal alopecia, periodic alopecia

Conditions Most Often Involving the Neck Region

Parasites: flea infestation, tick infestation, cuterebriasis
Neoplasia: basal-cell tumor, hemangioma, malignant fibrous histiocytoma, apocrine cyst, intracutaneous cornifying epithelioma, lipoma
Other: dermoid sinus, dermatitis herpetiformis

Conditions Most Often Involving the Topline

Parasites: fleas, lice, cheyletiellosis
Microbes: bacterial folliculitis, dermatophytosis
Endocrine: hypothyroidism, hyperadrenocorticism, growth hormone-responsive dermatosis
Neoplasia: apocrine adenoma, trichoepithelioma, pilomatrixoma, intracutaneous cornifying epithelioma, dermoid sinus, hepatoid-gland tumor
Other: vitamin A-responsive dermatosis, Dalmatian bronzing syndrome, nodular panniculitis, sebaceous adenitis, lupoid dermatosis, metabolic dermatoses, dermatitis herpetiformis

Conditions Most Often Involving the Underside

Parasites: sarcoptic mange, Pelodera dermatitis, trombiculiasis, dracunculiasis
Microbes: bacterial folliculitis, atypical mycobacteriosis, actinomycotic and eumycotic mycetoma
Immune: allergic inhalant dermatitis, contact dermatitis, erythema multiforme
Neoplasia: lipoma, liposarcoma
Other: calcinosis cutis, generic dog food disease, eosinophilic granuloma, lichenoid dermatoses

Conditions Most Often Involving the Genitalia

Neoplasia: melanoma, vascular nevi, squamous-cell carcinoma, transmissible venereal tumor, genital neoplasms, Sertoli-cell tumor, seminoma, interstitial-cell tumor, malignant histiocytosis
Other: estrogen-responsive disorders, hyperestrogenism, metabolic dermatoses

Conditions Most Often Involving the Legs

Parasites: demodicosis, sarcoptic mange, cutaneous dirofilariasis, dracunculiasis
Bacteria: callus pyoderma, actinomycotic mycetoma
Fungi: sporotrichosis, blastomycosis
Neoplasia: fibroma, fibrosarcoma, lipoma, hemangiopericytoma, hemangioma, histiocytoma, malignant fibrous histiocytoma, mast-cell tumor, collagenous nevi,
nodular dermatofibrosis, squamous-cell carcinoma, transmissible venereal tumor,
pilomatrixoma
Other: zinc-responsive dermatosis, calcinosis circumscripta, generic dog food disease,
spiculosis, acral lick dermatitis, acral mutilation syndrome, erythema multiforme,
dermatitis herpetiformis

Conditions Most Often Involving the Feet

Parasites: demodicosis, ticks, trombiculiasis, Pelodera dermatitis, hookworm dermatitis
Microbes: interdigital pyoderma, eumycotic mycetoma, blastomycosis, candidiasis,
furunculosis, bacterial granuloma, dermatophytosis
Immune: allergic inhalant dermatitis, food allergy, contact dermatitis, pemphigus
vulgaris, cutaneous vasculitis, drug eruption
Neoplasia: squamous-cell carcinoma, papilloma, melanoma, pilar cysts
Other: sterile pyogranuloma, foreign body reaction, lethal acrodermatitis, immuno-
deficiency, acral mutilation syndrome

Conditions Most Often Involving the Footpads

Parasites: hookworm dermatitis, Pelodera dermatitis
Microbes: dermatophytosis, intermediate systemic mycoses
Immune: pemphigus foliaceus, pemphigus erythematosus, lupus erythematosus, contact dermatitis
Neoplasia: pagetoid reticulosis, eccrine adenoma, eccrine adenocarcinoma, squamous-
cell carcinoma
Other: zinc-responsive dermatoses, generic dog food disease, tyrosinemia, nasodigital
hyperkeratosis, acral mutilation syndrome, lethal acrodermatitis, superficial
necrolytic dermatitis (metabolic dermatoses), foreign body penetration, epidermolysis bullosa simplex, familial vasculopathy

Conditions Most Often Involving
the Nails and Nail Beds

Microbes: bacterial paronychia, dermatophytosis, candidal paronychia, sporotrichosis,
blastomycosis, coccidioidomycosis
Immune: pemphigus vulgaris, lupus erythematosus, bullous pemphigoid, cutaneous
vasculitis, lupoid dermatosis, erythema multiforme, drug eruption
Other: demodicosis, nutritional imbalances, cardiopulmonary disease, lethal acrodermatitis

Conditions Most Often Involving the Mucocutaneous Junctions

Immune: pemphigus vulgaris, bullous pemphigoid, cicatricial pemphigoid, systemic lupus erythematosus, Vogt-Koyanagi-Harada-like syndrome, vitiligo, Sjögren's syndrome, erythema multiforme, drug eruption

Other: candidiasis, melanoma, fibrous histiocytoma (see also oral, periocular, and nasal tumors)

Conditions More Common in Males than Females

Neoplasia: testicular tumors, hemangiosarcoma, perianal-gland adenoma, perianal-gland adenocarcinoma, malignant histiocytosis, liposarcoma, B-cell lymphoma, melanoma, vascular nevi, cutaneous papilloma, apocrine adenoma, intracutaneous cornifying epithelioma

Other: acne, growth hormone-responsive dermatosis, eosinophilic granuloma, spiculosis

Conditions More Common in Females than Males

Neoplasia: fibrosarcoma, hemangiopericytoma, apocrine adenocarcinoma of anal sac origin, fibroma, lipoma

Other: estrogen-responsive dermatosis, hyperestrogenism, vulvar fold pyoderma, discoid lupus erythematosus, focal mucinosis

Conditions More Common in Younger Dogs

Parasites: demodicosis, cheyletiellosis, otodectic mange (ear mites)

Microbes: viral papillomatosis, acne, impetigo, dermatophytosis

Immune: allergic inhalant dermatitis, food allergy, Vogt-Koyanagi-Harada-like syndrome

Neoplasia: histiocytoma, sebaceous nevi, epidermal nevi, fibrous histiocytoma, intracutaneous cornifying epithelioma

Inherited: color mutant alopecia, cutaneous asthenia, dermatomyositis, epidermolysis bullosa simplex, ichthyosis

Other: zinc-responsive dermatosis, growth hormone-responsive dermatosis, dermoid sinus, albinism, vitiligo, tyrosinase deficiency, follicular dysplasia, spiculosis, eosinophilic granuloma, acral mutilation syndrome, lethal acrodermatitis, juvenile cellulitis, juvenile panniculitis, lichenoid dermatoses, sebaceous adenitis, sterile pyogranuloma, tyrosinemia

APPENDIX B

DIAGNOSTIC TESTS
USED IN DERMATOLOGY

Dermatology is a medical science that is often confusing to veterinarians and owners alike because so many different diseases, with different causes and different treatments, may look alike. Because there are so many look-alike diseases, diagnostic testing is very important. It is only by making an absolute diagnosis that treatment can be commenced with some certainty as to the likelihood of response. The alternative is that various treatments be tried, one after another, and this provides a service to no one.

SKIN SCRAPINGS
Skin scrapings are the most common diagnostic test performed in veterinary dermatology but they are often confusing to owners. A scalpel blade or similar instrument (the duller the better) is moistened with mineral oil and used to scrap away some of the surface epidermis in which may reside a number of different parasites. The scraping tool is then wiped onto a clean microscope slide and a microscope used to scan the slide for parasites. Skin scraping is therefore a quick and sometimes very rewarding procedure if parasites can be found. If no parasites are found, however, it does not mean that the problem is not caused by parasites. A negative skin scraping only means that parasites weren't present in the small area sampled.

Some parasites are easier to locate with scrapings than others. For example, the scabies mite is very difficult to recover, even with multiple scrapings. Demodex mites are often the easiest to find but still may occasionally be missed on scrapings.

Cheyletiella (walking dandruff) mites are often intermediates, being easy to find sometimes and difficult to find at other times.

Skin scrapings can also be used as part of a "yeast prep" to identify yeasts (especially *Malassezia pachydermatitis*) in surface scale. Special stains need to be applied to the sample to highlight the yeast and permit diagnosis.

BACTERIAL CULTURE AND SENSITIVITY

A bacterium is a very tiny organism which can either be beneficial to the animal (e.g., aid in digestion), be harmless (saprophytic), or produce disease (pathogenic). It is also important to remember that the surface of the skin is not sterile; the skin has its own normal community of microbes which form part of the surface landscape.

When a bacterial skin disease is suspected, samples are often collected to identify the type of bacteria involved and the best treatments available. This procedure is referred to as a bacterial culture and sensitivity. The culture refers to the process of growing the bacteria in the laboratory and the sensitivity is determined by exposing those bacteria to small doses of antibiotic to see which works best. This procedure requires about 18–24 hours of laboratory time to allow the bacteria to grow and to respond to the antibiotic challenge.

This sounds like a simple and very accurate test, but there are some problems. Since the surface of the skin has a normal population of microbes, contamination is a very critical issue. Almost any swab taken from inflamed skin will grow staphylococcal bacteria; that doesn't mean they are at the root of the problem. Therefore, samples need to be collected aseptically (without contamination). This often requires biopsies or removing pus from an intact pustule (pimple) with a syringe and needle.

A second pitfall is that the susceptibility information provided is based on the antibiotic concentration in the bloodstream. This doesn't take into account the situation if topical treatment is to be used (e.g., antibiotic ear drops) or if the antibiotics actually have difficulty reaching the microbes (e.g., with abscesses and granulomas). Other antibiotics may not be capable of penetrating from the bloodstream to the skin surface in an adequate concentration to exert any truly anti-bacterial action.

Therefore, bacterial cultures and sensitivities are important tests but must not be considered foolproof. They provide useful information but the results require careful evaluation and interpretation.

FUNGAL DIAGNOSTIC TESTS

Many different types of yeasts and fungi are present in the environment and on the skin surface, and not all result in skin disease. To help identify fungi that may contribute to skin disease, several tests are utilized.

The Wood's lamp is a special "black light" that causes some ringworm fungi to glow with a green color. It is not useful for other fungi and yeasts and only helps identify dermatophytes in perhaps 40% of cases. Actually, of the three main species of ringworm fungus, only one, *Microsporum canis,* glows at all and even then, less than 50% of the time. Because it is not a specific test, a positive Wood's lamp examination cannot confirm a diagnosis with any real accuracy and a negative test does not mean that ringworm fungi are not present.

Fungal and yeast "preps" are done by collecting hair and surface scale and examining them with a microscope. Special stains are often added to help highlight the organisms, which might be difficult to find. In people, this is known as a KOH (potassium hydroxide) preparation. With an experienced person at the microscope, this may be diagnostic about 60% of the time.

Fungal cultures are used to identify a variety of microbes that may be responsible for causing fungal infection in animals. The most common fungal infection is dermatophytosis (ringworm) and special fungal cultures have been developed (dermatophyte test medium or DTM) to help isolate and identify these organisms. Ringworm-causing fungi (dermatophytes) grow as white fluffy colonies in 3–14 days and frequently turn the color of the medium from yellow to red. The fungi can then be positively identified by microscopic examination. A diagnosis of dermatophytosis (ringworm) should not be made simply because the medium changes color. This color change is helpful but is not diagnostic.

To diagnose intermediate or deep (systemic) fungal infections, biopsies, blood tests, or cultures are used. These cultures should be performed at a diagnostic laboratory because of the risk to personnel in dealing with these microbes.

ALLERGY TESTING

Allergy testing is performed in a manner modified from the human procedure. In people, "pricks" are often made up the arms or across the back, but in animals the testing is done on the side of the chest. That area of the chest is shaved, and marks are made on the skin surface in a specific order to identify the substances to be injected. The "pricks" consist of the substances that are responsible for inhalant allergies, including tree, grass, and weed pollens, molds, house dust, house dust mites, feathers, and danders. To be reliable, at least 30 different substances should be tested and often many more than that are actually used. After each of these substances has been injected into the dermis in turn, the results are evaluated in about 15–20 minutes. Positive reactions consist of hives (wheals) at the site of injection. The interpretation is made by comparing the height, diameter, and redness of the reactions with two controls, a positive (e.g., histamine; 48/80), which gives a large reaction, and a negative (e.g., saline; sterile water), which gives no reaction. The entire test can be conducted in less than one hour. Some items (e.g., flea, staphylococcal bacteria, hormones) that may be used in testing sometimes do not show reactions for 48 hours.

Allergy testing is not foolproof and it is important that dogs not have corticosteroids, hormones, antihistamines, or specific tranquilizers in their system at the time of the test or they will interfere with the results. The amount of time one must wait between discontinuing drugs and testing is different for each different drug. If injectable corticosteroids were used, it may take months for all of the drug to get out of the system. For most of the regular antihistamines, a ten-day withdrawal time is adequate.

Recently, blood tests have become available for diagnosing allergies and these are referred to as in vitro allergy tests. Two technologies have been used in these tests: one is the ELISA (enzyme linked immunosorbent assay) and the other the RAST (radioallergosorbent test). These tests are not as accurate because they only measure the presence of an antibody in the bloodstream, not in the skin. They are useful when skin testing is not available, when an owner won't allow the fur to be shaved, or if the skin is too inflamed to permit testing. It must be cautioned that these tests provide only a laboratory result, not a diagnosis.

Patch testing is a different form of testing than intradermal allergy testing and is used to identify contact allergies and irritations. Unlike the intradermal test, which can be completed in less than one hour, this test takes 48 hours. Various substances including ground cover, leather, plastics, carpeting, etc., are applied to the skin surface and kept bandaged there for 48 hours. When the bandage is removed, the area is examined to see if the skin is inflamed where any of the substances were applied. This is a very difficult test to perform in dogs because the kits that are standardized for people are geared more to jewelry, clothing, and perfumes than to items in the environment. A canine kit must be assembled that is unique to each dog and the environment in which it lives.

BIOPSIES FOR HISTOPATHOLOGY

Biopsy for histopathology (microscopic tissue evaluation) is an important diagnostic tool in veterinary medicine but especially in dermatology since the tissue to be sampled (skin) is so readily accessible. Most of the new diseases that have been described in the past 20 years owe their identification and characterization to biopsy and histopathological evaluation by pathologists.

For the most part, biopsy is a simple procedure that can be frequently done with local anesthesia. Appropriate areas of the skin are selected, local anesthetic is injected into those areas, and within a minute or so samples can be collected by special "punches" or with a scalpel blade. The punches can take a core sample right through to the subcutaneous fat and the small hole remaining can be easily closed with one or two stitches. The biopsy samples are then placed in formalin (formaldehyde) and sent to pathologists for interpretation. Whenever possible, samples should be sent to pathologists with special expertise in skin problems.

When the pathologists receive the samples, they must be processed before they can be examined. They are cut to a proper shape, embedded in paraffin wax, and then cut again into very thin slices that will fit on a microscope slide. The slide is then subjected to a series of special stains before it is ready for examination. In a properly taken biopsy, all aspects of the skin should be available for evaluation: the epidermis, the dermis, and the panniculus.

The histopathology report provides a description of the changes seen in the skin, a morphologic diagnosis (based on pattern), and, when possible, an absolute diagnosis. Even if a full diagnosis cannot be made on the biopsy samples submitted, there is still much value in the exercise. Histopathology reports are never "negative." They provide a picture of the changes seen in a very small area of skin at a specific point in time. Sometimes they are valuable because of what they don't find and sometimes they can be "consistent with" a diagnosis but not be able to confirm it entirely.

The process can be compared to using photographs to identify people or things. Imagine a photograph of a bird. A gifted naturalist may be able to tell you a lot about the bird based on the material provided. There may not be enough evidence present to categorically name the species, but most can probably tell you what family it belongs to (e.g., sparrow, robin, crow). A car buff may be able to identify a car from one photo, but even if all the distinguishing features are not present, they could probably tell you the manufacturer, and perhaps the model or age. Skin biopsies are no different. We send samples to the pathologist to provide us as much information as possible on what's going on, based on small samples of skin tissue. Therefore, multiple biopsies of different stages greatly increase the chances of finding diagnostic changes. Biopsies are valuable diagnostic tools indeed, but should not be expected to tell the entire story. They will reveal the changes seen in a small region of skin surface at a particular point in time.

BIOPSIES FOR IMMUNOPATHOLOGY

Biopsies for immunopathology are used to help identify immunologic diseases by providing proof that antibodies are localizing in the skin. Although they are sometimes useful, they are not nearly as reliable in dogs as they are in people. In fact, even in dogs with confirmed immune-mediated skin diseases, only about 60% will have positive immunopathologic tests. These tests may therefore be helpful in confirming a diagnosis if the rest of the evidence is inconclusive, but a negative test means very little indeed.

Immunopathology includes direct immunofluorescence testing (DIT) and immunoperoxidase testing and is used to identify the presence of autoantibodies and/or complement in tissue. Most biopsy samples are stored in Michel's solution, rather than formalin, because formalin can destroy antibody in tissue. Immunoperoxidase studies can be performed on tissue fixed with formalin, but this form of testing is not widely available at this time. These tests are used to help diagnose pemphigus, lupus erythematosus, pemphigoid, cutaneous vasculitis, and dermatitis herpetiformis.

Indirect immunofluorescence testing is designed to detect disease-specific antibodies circulating in the blood. It is very useful in people, especially for detecting pemphigus autoantibody in the blood, but it has not proved reliable when used on dogs. While 90% of people have circulating pemphigus autoantibodies, less than 5% of dogs with pemphigus do. Therefore, this test is not recommended for use in dogs.

CYTOLOGY

Cytology (cyt- means cell and -ology means study of) is the study of free cells from tissues. Literally, it is a procedure used to try to make a diagnosis from the collection of a few cells rather than a whole biopsy. It is a quick procedure, relatively painless, and does not even require local anesthesia. The drawback is that some things are easier to diagnose than others with this procedure.

There are many ways cell collection can be accomplished. A "fine needle aspirate" involves sticking a needle with attached syringe into a tissue, applying gentle suction, and collecting some cells in the needle itself. The material is then expressed onto a clean microscope slide and often stained to help provide proper contrast. In dermatology, this procedure is most commonly utilized to evaluate lumps present on or beneath the skin.

An "impression smear" is performed by touching a microscope slide to the tissue being evaluated. The microscope slides may then be stained with a number of products to highlight certain cell types and products. This is a handy procedure to use with suspected infections, especially if intact pustules are available or scabs can be removed to provide an oozing surface. Alternatively, if a biopsy has already been taken, an impression smear can be made by touching the biopsy sample to a microscope slide — sometimes a quick diagnosis is possible, especially with tumors.

The advantage of cytology is that it is quick and that it may provide useful information. The disadvantage is that some diseases don't give up their cells as readily as others and that individual cells collected do not provide information on the "architecture" of the actual skin disease. Cytology is a valuable diagnostic aid but cannot provide the same depth of information as can biopsy.

HEMATOLOGY

Hematology is the study of blood cells. One of the most common blood tests performed in veterinary medicine is the complete blood count (CBC). This provides information about the red blood cells (erythrocytes), the white blood cells (leukocytes), and the clotting particles (platelets). This is not a specific test for skin diseases but provides some valuable clues as to what is going on in the body.

For instance, the white blood cell counts are elevated with a variety of infections, but low white counts usually suggest an immune deficiency. There are several types of white blood cells (e.g., lymphocytes, neutrophils, monocytes, etc.) and each has a job to do. Their evaluation therefore provides important information. If the red blood cells are lower than normal (anemia) this may also be associated with a variety of conditions. For example, anemia may be noted in conditions as varied as hypothyroidism and lupus erythematosus. Finally, there are also a number of disorders that cause platelet counts to drop.

Therefore, although blood counts rarely provide a diagnosis in dogs with skin diseases, they do provide information that should be considered.

BIOCHEMICAL PROFILES

Biochemical profiles, like blood counts, rarely diagnose skin diseases specifically, but provide useful information as to what is going on in the major organs of the body. Most profiles consist of a series of tests that measure liver and kidney function, pancreatic enzymes, proteins, blood sugar (glucose), cholesterol, and others. They help provide information to determine if the skin disease has effects inside the body, as well as outside.

IMMUNOLOGIC TESTS

There is no single test that provides us with insight as to immune status in the dog. Therefore, we rely on a series of different tests to help fill in the blanks and provide an overall picture of the immune health of an animal.

Some tests used to evaluate the immune system have already been discussed. Blood counts may provide a wealth of information if white blood cells (particularly lymphocytes or neutrophils) are lower than normal. Biochemical profiles often provide not only total protein levels, but the proportion of that total that are globulins, the fraction containing antibodies. Immunopathology is used in suspected immune-mediated skin diseases, to see if antibodies are actually being deposited in tissue.

Immunoglobulin tests are performed to see if animals with recurrent infections have normal amounts of the different classes of immunoglobulins, the family of substances to which antibodies belong. Immunoglobulin A (IgA) deficiency is the most common deficiency syndrome in dogs and many breeds are affected. A usual immunoglobulin profile includes levels for IgA, IgG, and IgM. Blood tests for allergies measure relative levels of specific IgE antibodies that can sometimes be helpful in the diagnosis of inhalant allergies.

Lymphocyte stimulation is a crude way to evaluate how the T-lymphocyte system is working. A blood sample is collected and the lymphocytes are exposed to chemicals (e.g., concavalin A, phytohemagglutin). How well the lymphocytes "stimulate" is a rough measure of their response to foreign material. A sample collected from a normal dog should be submitted at the same time, for comparison purposes.

Lymphocyte subsets, especially measurements of T-helper and T-suppressor lymphocytes, have recently become available by monoclonal antibody technology. At this point in time, these tests are not routinely available to veterinarians but are used for research purposes. The ratio of T-helper to T-suppressor cells can be calculated from these data and provides a useful measure of this aspect of the immune system.

Titers provide a rough measure of antibody levels to specific entities that may be viral, bacterial, fungal, or immunologic in origin. They are prepared by diluting the blood serum and exposing these dilutions to known amounts of the agent being tested for. For example, if the blood is mixed 50/50 with saline, this is a 1:2 dilution. If that sample is then mixed 50/50 with saline, there is now a 1:4 dilution. Obviously, if a reaction is noted at even high dilutions of serum, there must be very high levels of that specific antibody in the bloodstream. Thus, a titer of 1:64 reveals a much higher concentration of antibodies than does a titer of 1:8. Experience has taught us that each disease in which titers are helpful has a level that indicates likely problems. For example, most dogs with systemic fungal infections (e.g., coccidioidomycosis) have titers of 1:16 or greater. It is not unusual to find dogs that don't have the disease but have been previously exposed to have titers of 1:4 or less. Dogs with titers of 1:8 are usually considered "suspicious." Thus, titers provide important clues to diagnosis, but proper interpretation is critical.

The antinuclear antibody (ANA) test is used to measure the presence in the blood of antibodies directed against cell nuclei. These abnormal antibodies may target a variety of different tissues. Although the test was designed to diagnose lupus erythematosus, it may be positive in a number of other conditions and therefore should not be considered diagnostic on its own. The value is normally expressed as a titer that represents a concentration of antibody in the blood. In man, the concept of antinuclear antibodies has been carried to the next logical step, measuring antibodies to Sm antigen, histones, ribonucleoprotein (RNP), single-stranded DNA, PM-1, Jo-1, etc., to narrow down the possibilities of diagnosis as much as possible. Veterinary applications of these different ANAs are still in their infancy but will undoubtedly become available at some point in the future.

The LE (lupus erythematosus) cell test is one in which blood is collected, shaken gently to slightly damage cells, and then examined to see if autoantibodies prey on these disabled cells. When other white blood cells swallow the damaged nuclei they become known as LE cells, and are seen in about 60% of animals with systemic lupus erythematosus. Positive LE cell tests have been reported in many other conditions as well and this test is considered too subjective and not sensitive enough to be recommended as a confirming diagnostic test for lupus erythematosus.

Circulating immune complexes (CICs) are collections of antibodies and their targets that tend to float in the bloodstream and are occasionally deposited in tissue. Obviously, if these complexes are large enough they can cause damage by collecting in small blood vessels or in tissues, including the skin. Preliminary research suggests that dogs with lupus erythematosus, generalized demodicosis, dermatomyositis, cutaneous vasculitis, rheumatoid arthritis, systemic fungal infections, and pyoderma have significantly higher CICs than do normal dogs.

HAIR ANALYSIS

Hair analysis tends to wax and wane in popularity over the years, but there is little evidence that this procedure is helpful in diagnosing skin diseases, other than those caused by poisonings. It is common knowledge that mineral and trace element analysis of hair samples does not provide a reliable estimate of nutritional status. There is also no absolute correlation between hair levels of elements and levels in other body tissues, such as the liver or kidney. Finally, there is no standardization of what is so-called "normal" for hair mineral levels in man, and certainly not in animals. Hair analysis may have some validity, but, on its own, it is unlikely to provide enough information to allow a diagnosis to be made.

APPENDIX C

TREATMENTS USED IN DERMATOLOGY

MEDICATIONS USED TO TREAT PARASITES

Pyrethrins are natural insecticides derived from certain species of chrysanthemums. They are very effective insecticides for fleas and offer very little toxicity to mammals. Although they are relatively safe, the pyrethrins are degraded rapidly in the environment, especially in sunlight, and therefore give very little residual effect. Pyrethrin-based flea/tick dips may last for up to two weeks. Micro-encapsulation of the product allows for slow release of the pyrethrins and these provide suitable environmental control for up to two weeks.

Pyrethroids (synthetic pyrethrins) are similar to the natural pyrethrins, although safety and toxicity are more variable. Resistance is seen more commonly to the pyrethroids than to the pyrethrins.

Carbamates have good residual effect, are not broken down by sunlight, and the toxicity varies considerably between products. Carbamates are toxic by virtue of their ability to block an enzyme (acetylcholinesterase), which is important in nerve transmission. This feature is shared with the organophosphate insecticides. Signs of toxicity in an animal (e.g., pinpoint pupils, vomiting, diarrhea, seizures, etc.) should be treated as an emergency.

Organophosphates are considered to be one of the most toxic insecticides to mammals. As a group, their residual activity varies with the chemical structure from slight to very persistent. Commercially available organophosphates may be given orally, such as cythioate (e.g., Proban: Haver/Mobay), dabbed on the skin, such as fenthion (Prospot: Haver/Mobay), sprayed into the environment, such as dursban (e.g., Duratrol: 3M), used as a topical dip, such as phosmet (e.g., Paramite: Vet-Kem), or allowed to vaporize in a room, such as dichlorvos (e.g., Vapona: Shell). Malathion is a form of organophosphate that has fairly low toxicity but also only fair residual activity. Like the carbamates, organophosphates block the enzyme acetylcholinesterase and can very definitely result in toxicities if not carefully handled.

Insect Growth Regulators (IGRs) are not insecticides at all but rather hormone-like compounds which interrupt the development of the flea larva to adulthood. The most common products used are fenoxycarb and methoprene. Indoors they are very residual and persist for 75–90 days. Because they are not insecticides, there are few concerns about toxicity. The drawback is that since the product is not an insecticide it will not kill adult fleas, only prevent adults from developing from eggs and larvae already in the environment.

Ivermectin is a derivative of an organism found growing in the soil that has been found effective in the treatment of many internal and external parasites. Unfortunately, there is little effect on fleas or demodectic mange mites. Happily, there is quite a profound effect on Cheyletiella, Sarcoptes, and Otodectes (ear) mites. Currently, it is not licensed for this use in dogs and cats but has been found to be quite a safe compound, except in the Collie and its crosses, in which it appears to be profoundly toxic, to the point that animals have actually died from its use. A related cousin, milbemycin oxime (Interceptor) has been licensed as a heartworm preventive and has also demonstrated some effectiveness in the treatment of demodectic mange.

Amitraz is an antiparasitic dip marketed for the treatment of generalized demodectic mange (Mitaban: Upjohn) as well as in collar form for tick control (Preventic: Virbac). Amitraz is a useful product for demodicosis, but not one that effects cures in all cases. To be used effectively, the fur should be clipped to facilitate penetration of the drug, the animal must not be rinsed following the dip, and must not be allowed to get wet between dips. Dips are generally repeated every two weeks until the condition has been adequately controlled. The product has also been used successfully in the treatment of sarcoptic mange and is licensed for this purpose in Canada. Amitraz is effective in tick control because it prevents ticks from attaching to the skin and causes ticks already there to detach within 48 hours. One collar is effective for up to four months. This is an important breakthrough because this not only gets rid of ticks, but helps prevent a variety of diseases carried by those ticks, such as Lyme disease, ehrlichiosis, Rocky Mountain spotted fever, and babesiosis.

MEDICATIONS USED TO TREAT BACTERIAL INFECTIONS

Antibiotics are a group of chemicals that exert a harmful effect on certain micro-organisms. Some antibiotics are bactericidal (destroy bacteria), others bacteriostatic (inhibit growth of bacteria), and some may be either depending upon the concentration of the antibiotic.

The **beta-lactam** group of antibiotics includes penicillins and cephalosporins, important compounds not only in veterinary medicine but in human medicine as well. They act by killing bacteria and do this effectively in most skin infections. Most of the bacteria that cause skin infections in dogs are resistant to the basic penicillins (e.g., ampicillin, amoxicillin), so potentiated penicillins are often selected (e.g., oxacillin, cloxacillin, or amoxicillin combined with clavulanic acid) instead. Most of the cephalosporins (e.g., cephalexin, cephadroxil, cephradine) are quite effective in managing staphylococcal skin infections. New generations of cephalosporins and penicillins are constantly being formulated as organisms become resistant to existing varieties.

Aminocyclitol antibiotics, also known as **aminoglycosides,** include a large number of antibiotics, including streptomycin, gentamicin, neomycin, kanamycin, amikacin, and tobramycin. They are very effective at killing bacteria but are rarely used for skin infections because they can be toxic with long-term use. These antibiotics are therefore usually only prescribed for dermatology use in the form of topical solutions to be applied to the surface of the skin where the risk of toxic side effects is greatly reduced. They are also commonly found in ear drops but can cause damage there (ototoxicity) if used repeatedly.

Combinations of **trimethoprim** and **sulfonamides** (such as sulfamethoxazole, sulfadimethoxine, or sulfadiazine) kill bacteria effectively and potentiate the effects of one another. Side effects are few but include a slight risk of decreased tear production (keratoconjunctivitis sicca); this has not been as pronounced with a newer formulation of sulfadimethoxine and ormethoprim (Primor). Doberman Pinschers appear overly prone to side effects with sulfas and this drug should be cautiously used in the breed.

Macrolides such as erythromycin and lincosamides such as lincomycin and clindamycin are bacteriostatic antibiotics that are frequently prescribed for skin infections in dogs. A cousin, clindamycin (Antirobe: Upjohn) is used for the treatment of deep infected wounds or abscesses in the dog.

Chloramphenicol is a bacteriostatic antibiotic that is commonly prescribed to animals, but humans seem to have an intolerance for the product and often experience a number of unacceptable side effects. Dogs are not nearly as prone to these side effects and chloramphenicol is usually successful in the treatment of simple bacterial infections, but the creation of resistant organisms poses an ever-increasing problem.

Fluoroquinolones have only recently become common antibiotics used in dogs. Products like enrofloxacin (Baytril: Haver/Mobay) reach blood levels quickly and kill bacteria rapidly. Other examples include ciprofloxacin (Cipro) and norfloxacin (Noroxin). Only Baytril is licensed for use in dogs. It should not be used in young, actively growing dogs because it may adversely affect developing cartilage.

Table 1. Examples of Antibiotics

FAMILY	GENERIC NAME	EXAMPLE
Penicillin	Amoxicillin	Amoxil
	Ampicillin	Amcil; Omnipen
	Cloxacillin	Orbenin; Tegopen
	Dicloxacillin	Dynapen
	Oxacillin	Prostaphlin
	Carbenicillin	Geopen
	Amoxicillin-clavulanate	Clavamox
Cephalosporin	Cefamandole	Mandrol
	Cefazolin	Kefzol
	Cephadroxil	Cefa-Tabs
	Cephalexin	Keflex
	Cephaloridine	Loridine
	Cephalothin	Keflin
	Cephapirin	Cefadyl
	Cephradine	Velosef
Aminoglycosides	Amikacin	Amiglyde-V
	Gentamicin	Gentocin
	Kanamycin	Kantrim
Trimethoprim-sulfa	Trimethoprim-sulfamethoxazole	Septra
	Trimethoprim-sulfadiazine	Tribrissen
	Ormethoprim-sulfadimethoxine	Primor
Fluoroquinolones	Ciprofloxacin	Cipro
	Enrofloxacin	Baytril
	Norfloxacin	Noroxin
Chloramphenicol	Chloramphenicol	Chloramphenicol
Macrolides	Erythromycin	Erythromycin
	Tylocin	Tylocine
	Vancomycin	Vancocin
Lincosamides	Lincomycin	Lincocin
	Clindamycin	Antirobe
Tetracyclines	Doxycycline	Vibramycin
	Minocycline	Minocin
	Oxytetracycline	Liquamycin
	Tetracycline	Panmycin

PRODUCTS USED TO TREAT FUNGAL INFECTIONS

Griseofulvin (e.g., Fulvicin) is a antifungal used in the treatment of ringworm (dermatophytosis). It is available in two forms. The microsize preparation must be given with a fat meal (e.g., corn oil), but this is not necessary for the ultra-microsize preparation. It is normally given for 6 weeks, but at least until two weeks beyond apparent clinical cure. The drug has an unpleasant taste and may cause vomiting in dogs. The product should not be given to pregnant animals, since it has been proven to cause birth defects.

Ketoconazole (e.g., Nizoral) is a broad-spectrum antifungal agent, administered orally and effective against dermatophytes (ringworm), Candida, and the systemic mycoses. There are few side effects, but liver function is usually monitored throughout therapy.

Amphotericin B (e.g., Fungizone) is a potent antifungal drug that must be given intravenously. Because of its many side effects (including kidney toxicity and anemia), it has largely been replaced by newer products. It is still used occasionally in patients that do not appear to benefit from ketoconazole. Treatment is often lengthy (months) and must continue for four weeks beyond clinical cure.

Flucytosine (Ancobon; Ancotil) is an oral antifungal agent useful in the treatment of cryptococcosis and candidiasis. It is less toxic than Amphotericin B but still has some mild adverse effects on the liver, bone marrow, and digestive tract. Its main limitation is that fungi quickly become resistant, sometimes in as little as three weeks.

IMMUNE STIMULANTS

Immune stimulants are used to bolster a faltering immune system so that the animal mounts its own natural assault on the disease process. How immune stimulants work and their actual effectiveness are somewhat controversial, but many animals do benefit. Most stimulants are given by injection, but some natural ones are given orally.

Products such as **Staphoid-AB** (Burroughs-Wellcome) and **Staphage lysate** (Delmont) are derived from staphylococcal bacteria and administered in the hopes of stimulating the immune system to functional levels. **ImmunoRegulin** (Immunovet) is derived from a different bacterium (Proprionibacterium acnes) and the company makes many claims for its effectiveness. One of its main drawbacks is that it needs to be injected intravenously, or directly into the abdominal cavity.

Autogenous bacterins are made from bacteria cultured from the dog's skin and grown in a laboratory. In theory, they should be very effective, since they are made from the strains of bacteria causing the problems, but this has not been proven.

Levamisole is marketed as a "wormer" in large animals but has been shown to also potentiate the immune system in carefully regulated dosages. Since it may also cause a number of worrying side effects, patients should be carefully monitored.

Some natural products that are purported to act as immune stimulants are **thymus gland extracts** and **dimethylglycine.** The rationale for using thymus gland extracts is that the thymus gland is the "master gland" of the immune system, producing several important hormones. This may have some merit, but too few cases have been evaluated to draw any valid conclusions.

CORTICOSTEROIDS

Corticosteroids are cortisone-like products which have an effect on most tissues in the body. They are excellent at reducing inflammation in the skin and other organs but have many side effects with long-term use. Dogs produce their own form of cortisone, called cortisol, in their adrenal glands, located at the top of the kidneys. If corticosteroids are administered to dogs, especially long-term, the body perceives this increased level and signals the adrenal glands to stop producing their own cortisol.

Thus, the adrenal glands may atrophy and be incapable of responding to the body's request for cortisol production. In the meantime, all of the other tissues of the body are subjected to the abnormally high levels of corticosteroids being administered. Recent research has shown that 5 weeks' worth of prednisone (in anti-inflammatory doses) will compromise adrenal function for 2 weeks.

Initial side effects seen are very common and include an increase in thirst (polydipsia), urination (polyuria), and hunger (polyphagia). These side effects are not dangerous in the short term, but are inconvenient. In time, corticosteroid use can cause diabetes mellitus, decreased resistance to infection, gastric ulcers, decreased thyroid and growth hormone levels, fluid retention, and the deposition of fat in the liver. Many other effects may also be seen and chronically elevated blood levels of corticosteroids results in a condition known as hyperadrenocorticism or Cushing's disease. Because of all of these potential side effects, corticosteroids should be cautiously administered, especially in the following situations: diabetes mellitus, pregnancy, young animals, epilepsy, heart or kidney disease, infectious diseases, osteoporosis, and gastro-intestinal ulcers.

Why, then, are corticosteroids so commonly prescribed? In proper doses and short durations, corticosteroids effectively suppress most forms of inflammation from the itching of allergies to the joint pain of arthritis. In the proper hands and with the proper respect, corticosteroids are an important tool in the management of many skin problems.

Whenever possible, alternate day therapy should be instituted so that the adrenal gland has an opportunity during the "off" day to produce some of its own cortisol, thus making adrenal atrophy a less likely possibility. Only certain corticosteroids may be used on an alternate day basis (e.g., prednisone, prednisolone, triamcinolone) and these should always be the first choice of therapy. Long-acting injectable forms of corticosteroid are less desirable.

Table 2. Examples of Oral Corticosteroids

ACTIVE FORM OF CORTICOSTEROID	EXAMPLES
Prednisone	Prednisone; Deltasone
Prednisolone	Prednisolone
Triamcinolone	Aristocort; Kenacort
Flumethasone	Flucort
Dexamethasone	Azium

ANTIHISTAMINES

The first antihistamine, Antergan, was marketed in France in 1942. Its first American counterpart, Benadryl (diphenhydramine hydrochloride), entered the picture two years later and now there are almost 200 brands of antihistamines on the market to choose from. Antihistamines tend to work well in about 30% of allergic dogs and, although this may not seem like a high percentage, they usually have very few side effects. Most of the "classic" antihistamines can make an animal drowsy, but they have few other risks. Some of the newer antihistamines, such as terfenadine (Seldane), are much less sedating.

The most commonly prescribed antihistamines for use in the dog are clemastine (Tavist), hydroxyzine (Atarax), diphenhydramine (Benadryl), and chlorpheniramine (Chlortrimeton). It is often necessary to try several different antihistamines in a dog to see if one will work. Each one should be given for at least a week before being discontinued.

Combinations of antihistamines with small amounts of prednisones (e.g., Temaril P, Vanectyl P, Cortabs) are a suitable compromise initially if dogs cannot be controlled entirely with antihistamine alone. In general, the dose of corticosteroid in the combination is quite low and is much safer than maintaining the dog on prednisone alone.

OMEGA-3 AND OMEGA-6 FATTY ACIDS
The omega 3 fatty acids include eicosapentaenoic acid (EPA), docosapentaenoic acid (DPA), and docosahexaenoic acid (DHA). These are long, awkward names, but all originate from plankton or algae that are then eaten by fish. Some fish (e.g., krill, herring, mackerel, and salmon) store these fatty acids in their muscles, while others (e.g., cod) store them in their livers. Cod liver oil is an excellent source of omega-3 fatty acids, but it is toxic in the amount needed to be effective in reducing inflammation. Their primary use to date has been in the treatment of allergic dermatitis in dogs.

The omega-6 fatty acids are derived from plants, including evening primrose oil, sunflower oil, and borage oil. They have also been shown to reduce inflammation in a natural way.

The success rate for controlling allergies in dogs with combinations of omega-3 and omega-6 fatty acids is perhaps 20%. This might not seem like a large percentage, but these products have few if any side effects. These essential fatty acids are more successful at curbing sores and infection associated with allergies than with itchiness. Most products currently available (Omega Pet, DermCaps; EFA-Z Plus) contain combinations of the omega-3 and omega-6 fatty acids. Single-purpose supplements are also available: Pet-F.A. contains omega-6 fatty acids and Nutrisol contains omega-3 fatty acids.

RETINOIDS
Retinoids are synthetic cousins of vitamin A and are used to treat acne and keratinization disorders in people. The most common retinoids available are isotretinoin (Accutane) and etretinate (Tegison). Neither are currently licensed to be used in dogs. Acitretin is another retinoid which is not yet available.

Etretinate has a more profound effect on surface epithelium and so has been used in the treatment of some keratinization disorders in dogs. Accutane has been used experimentally in the treatment of sebaceous adenitis, acne, and perianal fistulae.

Side effects of retinoid use are common in people and they should never be given to individuals that are pregnant. In dogs, side effects do not appear to be as prevalent, but lethargy, painful joints, itchiness, elevated triglyceride levels, and other problems have been encountered. Animals on retinoids should be carefully monitored with routine blood tests and radiographs (x-rays) if necessary.

CHEMOTHERAPY

Chemotherapy describes the use of chemicals to treat disease. In a loose sense, we reserve this term for drugs used to treat cancers and autoimmune diseases. Drugs that fall into this category that are used to treat skin diseases include azathioprine, six-mercaptopurine, cyclophosphamide, chlorambucil, doxorubicin, methotrexate, and vincristine.

Azathioprine (Imuran) is probably the most commonly prescribed chemotherapy in dogs, used for the treatment of a variety of autoimmune skin diseases. It doesn't start working immediately and takes 3–5 weeks before its beneficial effects are seen. It is relatively safe compared to other chemotherapies, but blood counts and liver function tests should be performed regularly to minimize the risk of serious side effects. Six-mercaptopurine, a by-product of azathioprine, can also be used in the treatment of autoimmune skin diseases and some cancers.

Cyclophosphamide (Cytoxan: Mead Johnson) and **chorambucil** (Leukeran: Burroughs-Wellcome) are alkylating agents used in cancer chemotherapy and only infrequently in the treatment of autoimmune diseases. Cyclophosphamide has a number of note-worthy side effects and routine monitoring is a critical part of treatment. Blood counts as well as liver and kidney function tests are indicated. Hair loss is seen most commonly in those breeds with continuous hair growth (e.g., Poodles, Old English Sheep-dogs, and Schnauzers) and the effects are often reversible on discontinuation of therapy. Chlorambucil is the least toxic drug in this class and is also useful in the treatment of autoimmune disorders, especially in small dogs.

Doxorubicin HCl (Adriamycin: Adria Laboratories) is useful in the treatment of many skin cancers. The drug is metabolized by the liver and excreted by the kidneys and the animal's urine may temporarily turn a red-orange color. It is administered intra-venously and toxicity to the heart is a very important adverse effect of this drug. An antihistamine is often given with the drug because another potential side effect is allergic reactions.

Methotrexate (Methotrexate: Lederle) is an antimetabolite and is most commonly used in the treatment of lymphoma. The vinca alkaloids vincristine and vinblastine are very uncommonly used in dermatology, even in the treatment of autoimmune skin diseases, but do find some application in the treatment of skin cancers.

CHRYSOTHERAPY

The use of gold compounds (chrysotherapy), either Solganal (aurothioglucose) or Myochrysine (gold sodium thiomalate) to treat autoimmune disease has become more routine over the last few years. Despite the fact that the active ingredient is indeed gold, treatment is not as expensive as one would think. An oral gold compound, tri-ethylphosphine gold (Aurinofin: SKF; Ridaura), is also available and is currently undergoing evaluation.

Therapy is initiated by giving two test doses a week apart by intramuscular injection. If there are no reactions, gold therapy is continued weekly until the condition is seen to respond, then tapered to alternate weeks, then monthly. Side effects are possible, so all patients have their blood and urine monitored prior to each injection.

DAPSONE

Dapsone is a sulfone used in people for the treatment of leprosy. Dapsone is used in veterinary medicine to treat a few conditions, namely cutaneous vasculitis, sub-corneal pustular dermatosis, and dermatitis herpetiformis. Since side effects are common with this drug, patients must be routinely monitored with blood tests.

PLASMAPHERESIS

Plasmapheresis, or plasma exchange, involves removing blood from a dog, filtering it, and then returning the filtered blood to the dog. It is very rarely used because it is very expensive, and available from only a few locations. It is used in the treatment of some immunologic diseases in people, as well as some cancers. In dogs, it has been used principally in the treatment of systemic lupus erythematosus (SLE), where antibody levels are quickly reduced in the blood. The procedure must be repeated several times to effectively reduce antibody levels and prednisone or other immuno-suppressive drugs must still be administered to prevent a rebound in antibody levels. Plasmapheresis does not cure the condition, it just temporarily reduces the antibody levels that are causing the problem.

CYCLOSPORINE A

Cyclosporine A is an important immunosuppressive agent used in tissue transplants. It has been successful in a small percentage of autoimmune skin diseases, but its current cost does not rationalize its use in most dogs where more effective treatments are available.

TOPICAL PRODUCTS

Topical preparations are those that are applied to the skin rather than being given internally. The basic rule to selecting topicals is: if the skin is wet, "dry it," and if the skin is dry, "wet it." In practical terms, this means to apply moisturizing products to dry skin and drying agents to skin that is weeping or moist. Creams and ointments lubricate the skin and form a protective covering that traps and holds in water as well as protecting it from the environment. It is not wise to apply creams and oint-ments to sores, or "hot spots," because infection can be sealed in as well as water. Lotions are liquids that contain suspended medicinal agents. They tend to be dry-ing, cooling, and helpful in relieving some itchiness. As such, they are ideally suited for oozing lesions that need to be dried up. Gels are clear, colorless substances that, when rubbed into the skin, are absorbed almost completely and are not overly messy to use.

Topical antibacterial agents such as neomycin, polymixin B, bacitracin, gramicidin, and nitrofurazone are commonly used in topical preparations and are useful for treat-ing very localized infections. If large areas of skin need to be treated for bacteria, topical antiseptics such as chlorhexidine, cetrimide, povidone-iodine, or benzoyl peroxides are much more practical.

Topical antifungal agents are commonly prescribed in human medicine, but because of the dense haircoat of animals, they are less suitable for use in dogs. Products like clotrimazole (e.g., Canesten; Lotrisone; Mycelex), miconazole (e.g., Conofite), econazole (e.g., Ecostatin; Spectazole), and ketoconazole (Nizoral) are effective against dermatophytes, Candida yeasts, and Malassezia (Pityrosporon) yeasts. Nystatin is commonly found in topical treatments, but is much more effective against Candida than Malassezia, and Malassezia is by far the most common yeast found on dog skin.

For more generalized antifungal treatment, chlorhexidine, povidone-iodine, captan, and lime sulfur are often used in baths or dips. Chlorhexidine is preferred because it is very effective and quite gentle on the skin. Both captan and lime sulfur are products marketed to control garden fungi but have been used for years, in diluted form, to treat ringworm. They are not without risk because capstan can cause contact sensitization in people and lime sulfur is often smelly and can stain the haircoat.

A new antifungal agent, enilconazole, is currently available in Europe as a dip and has been found to be quite effective in the treatment of dermatophytosis.

Topical corticosteroids are used to reduce inflammation in localized areas, but most products available are too potent for regular use. These products are designed to be used for only 7–10 days because, after about 2 weeks, the corticosteroid actually gets absorbed through the skin and causes effects internally. This has been demonstrated for many of the most popular topical corticosteroids, including triamcinolone acetonide (Panolog), dexamethasone (Tresaderm), betamethasone valerate (Topagen), and fluocinolone (Synotic). These products may be used for a week or so to bring the inflammation under control, but then it is important to consider safer products for long-term use. The safest corticosteroid for long-term use is hydrocortisone (e.g., Dermacool-HC; Cortispray; Cort-aid; Dermaguard).

Combinations of antibiotics and corticosteroids are often prescribed to treat ear problems (otitis externa), since both the inflammation and infection need to be addressed. They often work well for this purpose, but the most common products cannot be used long-term, principally because of their corticosteroid content. Also, with routine use they promote bacterial resistance to their antibiotic component. Examples include Tresaderm, Panolog, and Oribiotic.

Medicated shampoos are designed to remove scales, crusts, microbes, and debris from the skin surface and are often an important aspect of treatment. Medicated shampoos are designed to work on the skin surface, not the haircoat. Therefore, the shampoo must make contact with the skin for 5–15 minutes or as specified by the manufacturer. Although there are many more human shampoos available than veterinary products, it should be kept in mind that some major differences do exist between animal and human skin, not the least of which is that dogs have compound hair follicles and the pH of their skin (5.5–7.2) is less acidic than that of humans (5.5 average). The antiseborrheic shampoos are discussed in the chapter on keratinization disorders. Antiseborrheic ingredients include sulfur, salicylic acid, selenium sulfide, tar, and benzoyl peroxide.

Hypoallergenic shampoos are mild shampoos that lack many of the properties of medicated shampoos that may be irritating to a dog's skin. These shampoos are not designed for allergic animals, who frequently require medicated shampoos to help relieve their symptoms of itchiness and scaling. Hypoallergenic shampoos should be used on dogs with sensitive skin that do not require harsher medicated products.

Shampoos containing perfumes, astringents, and medicaments may be poorly tolerated by individuals with sensitive skin. Dishwashing detergents which contain emollients are often good products for being mild, cutting grease, and cleansing, but care should be taken when ethyl alcohol is a component, since dogs have apparently been poisoned by bathing with such products.

Moisturizers were designed to re-hydrate the skin in dry, scaly conditions or following shampooing with drying agents, such as benzoyl peroxide. Moisturizers may be applied directly to the coat (e.g., Humilac: Virbac; Hylyt efa: DVM) or applied as a final rinse following bathing (e.g., Alpha Keri; Skin-So-Soft). It is imperative that final rinses not be overdone since these products, if not diluted prooperly (e.g., 1 capful per gallon of water), will result in animals with slick, oily coats. Therefore, apply these agents in moderation.

ADDITIONAL READING

Ackerman, L.: *Practical Canine Dermatology*. American Veterinary Publications, Goleta, CA. 1989, 369 pp.

Ackerman, L.: Autoimmune disorders. In *Handbook of Small Animal Practice,* 2nd edition. R. Morgan (ed.). Churchill Livingstone, New York. 1992, 991–996.

Ackerman, L.: Hypersensitivity disorders. In *Handbook of Small Animal Practice,* 2nd edition. R. Morgan (ed.). Churchill Livingstone, New York. 1992, 996–999.

Ackerman, L.: Adverse reactions to foods. *Journal of Veterinary Allergy and Clinical Immunology,* 1993; 1(1): 18–22.

Ackerman, L.: Diagnosing inhalant allergies: Intradermal or in vitro testing? *Veterinary Medicine,* 1988; 83: 779–788.

Ackerman, L.: Medical and immunotherapeutic options for treating atopic dogs. *Veterinary Medicine,* 1988; 83: 790–797.

Ackerman, L.: Basic guide to the immune system. *Pet Focus,* 1991; 3(4): 7–9.

Bukowski, J.: Real and potential occupational health risks associated with insecticide use. *Compendium on Continuing Education for the Practicing Veterinarian,* 1990; 12(11): 1617–1626.

Campbell, K. L.; Small, E.: Identifying and managing the cutaneous manifestations of various endocrine diseases. *Veterinary Medicine,* 1991; 86: 118–135.

Campbell, K. L.; Uhland, C. F.; Dorn, G. P.: Effects of oral sunflower oil on serum and cutaneous fatty acid concentration profiles in seborrheic dogs. *Veterinary Dermatology,* 1992; 3(1): 29–35.

DeBoer, D. J.: Canine staphylococcal pyoderma: Newer knowledge and therapeutic advances. *Veterinary Medicine Report,* 1990; 2: 254–266.

Dodds, W. J.: Immune deficiency diseases. *Pet Focus,* 1991; 3(4): 10–12.

Foley, R. H.: Parasitic mites of dogs and cats. *Compendium on Continuing Education for the Practicing Veterinarian,* 1991: 13(5): 783–800.

Garris, G. I.: Control of ticks. *Veterinary Clinics of North America: Small Animal Practice,* 1991; 21(1): 173–183.

Hargis, A. M.; Mundell, A. C.: Familial canine dermatomyositis. *Compendium on Continuing Education for the Practicing Veterinarian,* 1992; 14(7): 855–864.

Kunkle, G. A.: Canine dermatomyositis: A disease with an infectious origin. *Compendium on Continuing Education for the Practicing Veterinarian,* 1992; 14(7): 866–871.

Medleau, L.; Chalmers, S. A.: Resolution of generalized dermatophytosis without treatment in dogs. *Journal of the American Veterinary Medical Association,* 1992; 201(12): 1891–1892.

Medleau, L.; White-Weithers, M. E.: Treating and preventing the various forms of dermatophytosis. *Veterinary Medicine,* 1992; 87: 1096–1100.

Merchant, S. R.; Taboada, J.: Dermatologic aspects of tick bites and tick-transmitted diseases. *Veterinary Clinics of North America: Small Animal Practice,* 1991; 21(1): 145–155.

Meyer, D. J.; Moriello, K. A.; Feder, B. M.; et al.: Effect of otic medications containing glucocorticoids on liver function test results in healthy dogs. *Journal of the American Veterinary Medical Association,* 1990; 196(5): 743–744.

Miller, Jr., W. H.: Topical management of seborrhea in dogs. *Veterinary Medicine,* 1990; 85: 122–131.

Miller, Jr., W. H.; Scott, D. W.; Buerger, R. G.; et al.: Necrolytic migratory erythema in dogs: A hepatocutaneous syndrome. *Journal of the American Animal Hospital Association,* 1990; 26(6): 573–581.

Miller, Jr., W. H.; Scott, D. W.; Scarlett, J. M.: Evaluation of an allergy screening test for use in atopic dogs. *Journal of the American Veterinary Medical Association,* 1992; 200(7): 931–935.

Moriello, K. A.: Dermatologic manifestations of internal and external parasitism. *Companion Animal Practice,* 1988; 2(3): 12–17.

Nelson, R. W.; Feldman, E. C.; Ford, S. L.: Topics in the diagnosis and treatment of canine hyperadrenocorticism. *Compendium on Continuing Education for the Practicing Veterinarian,* 1991; 13(12): 1797–1805.

Nesbitt, G. H.; Ackerman, L. J. (eds.): *Dermatology for the small animal practitioner.* Veterinary Learning Systems. 1991, 250 pp.

Panciera, D. L.: Canine hypothyroidism. Part II. Thyroid function tests and treatment. *Compendium on Continuing Education for the Practicing Veterinarian,* 1990; 12(6): 843–857.

Plant, J. D.; Rosenkrantz, W. S.; Griffin, C. E.: Factors associated with and prevalence of high Malassezia pachydermatis numbers on dog skin. *Journal of the American Veterinary Medical Association,* 1992; 201(6): 879–882.

Power, H. T.; Ihrke, P. J.; Stannard, A. A.; Backus, K. Q.: Use of etretinate for treatment of primary keratinization disorders (idiopathic seborrhea) in cocker spaniels, West Highland white terriers, and basset hounds. *Journal of the American Veterinary Medical Association,* 1992; 201(3): 419–429.

Roudebush, P.; Cowell, C. S.: Results of a hypoallergenic diet survey of veterinarians in North America with a nutritional evaluation of homemade diet prescriptions. *Veterinary Dermatology,* 1992; 3(1): 23–28.

Rudmann, D. G.; Coolman, B. R.; Perez, C. M.; Glickman, L. T.: Evaluation of risk factors for blastomycosis in dogs: 857 cases (1980–1990). *Journal of the American Veterinary Medical Association,* 1992; 201(11): 1754–1759.

Sosna, C. B.; Medleau, L.: The clinical signs and diagnosis of external parasite infestation. *Veterinary Medicine,* 1992; 87: 549–564.

Sosna, C. B.; Medleau, L.: Treating parasitic skin conditions. *Veterinary Medicine,* 1992; 87: 573–586.

White, S. D.; Rosychuk, R. A.; Reinke, S. I.; Paradis, M.: Use of tetracycline and niacinamide for treatment of autoimmune skin disease in 31 dogs. *Journal of the American Veterinary Medical Association,* 1992; 200(10): 1497–1500.

White, S. D.: Pododermatitis. *Veterinary Dermatology,* 1989; 1: 1–18.

INDEX